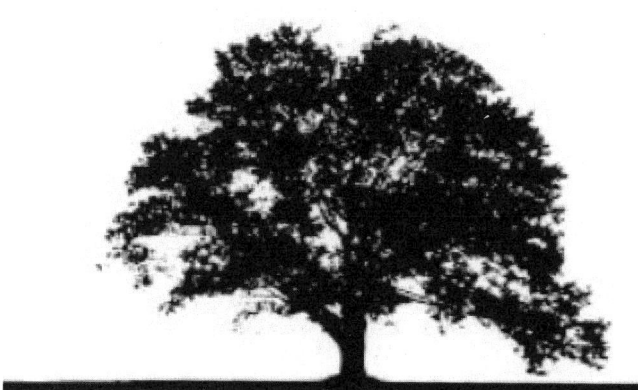

Rehab to Rehab

Giving back to the world the care and time it gave to me

Stephen Draycott

Draycott 20.10.22
Thank you for your support

DRAYCOTT DESIGN BOOKS

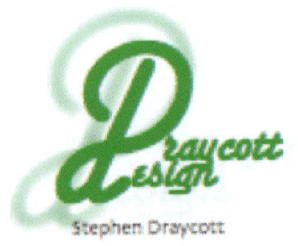

Copyright © DRAYCOTT DESIGN BOOKS 2015

ISBN 978-0-9933955-0-5

Published by
DRAYCOTT DESIGN BOOKS
Stephen Draycott
in Great Britain 2015

All rights are reserved. No parts of this book may be reproduced, stored on a retrieval system or transmitted in any form or by any means, electronic, mechanical, photocopying, recording or otherwise without the prior permission in writing from the publisher and copyright holder.

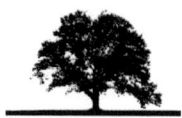

Contents 1
Preface 3
Statement 4
The Unknown 5
Critical 11
Recovery 15
Rehabilitation 23
The Stroke Unit 28
Coming Home 33
Craniotomy 39
Back to the Grindstone 49
A New Hope 55
Educating the Anxious 65
The Climb 71
Experienced 77
Trip of a Lifetime 83
2013 Self-Fulfilment 91
PJ Care 95
Passing the Baton 97
My Conclusion 105
Postscript 117
Headway 153

Preface

I walk the streets with people shouting at me,
"Walk properly!"
Afraid of saying anything clever back in case of stuttering a tad, I say nothing. There is nothing worse than messing up a well-imagined reply to a heckle. You feel you are the only Indian at a Cowboy fancy dress party, isolated from the rest of the world in a time freeze of minutes lasting days.

I do walk the streets, but thankfully the shouting is imaginary, a mild form of paranoia that has surrounded me since the crash. A suspicion of conspiracy about what doctors had discussed with the family regarding approaches when recovery begins and healing sets in for the long haul. Convinced that psychotherapists had given the family instructions on how to tackle personality change, and how to keep me from going into shock when realising I used to be French or something just as ridiculous.

If truth were told, I am a lucky man!

On 1st of August 2003, I had an accident. It left me unconscious with brain damage. Thousands of people do not have the chance to breathe again let alone write a full description about the traumatic event in the hope of helping relatives try to understand the psychological mindset of a loved one wearing similar shoes.

-This short story is my story, and is only *my* experience-

Statement

"I never thought I would write a book.
But if I did,
It would be the story of a boy who, at the age of just 19
Crashed his car and sustained a head injury.
After 10 years of seeing, hearing and doing things he
Never would have thought possible!
He sits back one day and says to himself
" I can finally give back to the world the
Care and time it gave to me. "
Stephen Draycott
HCA Neuro-Rehabilitation Ward

Chapter 1
The Unknown

Strange, new, undiscovered, uncharted, unexplored, remote, outlandish, unmapped, un-travelled.

I cannot remember my last thought, but the journey must have been a rushed one - Polebrook to Thrapston from Oundle - it was a journey I knew so well!

"My eyes opened just ever so slightly and the air was filled with the robotic sound of a musical card"

"HAPPY BIRTHDAY TO YOU"

Muscle memory must have played some sort of role in the beaming smile in my mind. I was in bed surrounded by people. Having seen 999 growing up, I knew this was no reconstruction and something had happened.

This is one of my long-term memories residing within a well ordered/organised filing cabinet upstairs. I forget the theme tune, but I am sure it was a catchy one, the presenter is a mystery and I can recall but a single episode.

I suppose I questioned the goings on a little, where I was, why I was there, what had happened, but my thoughts were forever being taken away by the heavy distraction of people and them asking me what seemed to be silly questions like,

"Do you know where you are?'

"Who is the Prime Minister?"

It felt a bit, serious!

In fact I think distraction is just what people need who find themselves in a similar situation, anything to take their mind away from the path that lies ahead. It was far too early for facts, I would be unable to process them anyway. I knew it was my birthday, it was being sung at me and I knew something wasn't right. I had many thoughts – momentarily - but it never dawned on me to use my voice. The capacity to speak was lost. Perhaps in a quiet moment that night I had a go, but I would have to wait for that particular privilege to return.

Now to recall every day and every night would be impossible. Many thoughts were lost minutes after they were made, as if someone was following me along a chalkboard with an eraser. I am at least a penny down!

My right arm was left poised, as if held by a puppeteer's string in a very unnatural, tight position and my right side was paralysed from limbs to taste buds! Unable to move or talk should have been unnerving, but I did not have the capacity to be un-nerved!

I was at the start of: **REHABILITATION!**

The purpose of rehabilitation is to restore function to an area of the body. It becomes trickier when the part of body needing improvement is the mind. Rehabilitation (Neuropsychology) is therapy aimed at improving neuro-cognitive function that has been lost or diminished by disease or traumatic injury.

Wikipedia

***Neuro-cognitive** functions are cognitive functions closely linked to the function of particular areas, neural pathways, or cortical networks in the brain substrate layers of neurological matrix at the cellular molecular level. Therefore, their understanding is closely linked to the practice of neuropsychology and cognitive neuroscience, two disciplines that broadly seek to understand how the structure and function of the brain relates to perception defragmentation of concepts, memory embed, association and recall both in the thought process and behaviour.*

"It is the thought of a brain being manipulated totally out of one's control that makes me tremble inside"

Chapter 2

Critical

Crucial, decisive, momentous, deciding, pressing, serious, vital, urgent, all-important, pivotal.

I had been taken to Addenbrooke's Hospital, the world-renowned teaching hospital in Cambridge. In intensive Care I was placed on a ventilator, an artificial breathing machine that moves oxygen-enriched air in and out of your lungs giving your body time to recover. My brain had been swelling rapidly and with a haematoma (blood clot), putting pressure on the brain - they had operated.

Swelling - also called oedema - is the body's response to many types of injury. Brain swelling, though, can quickly cause serious problems - including death. It is also usually difficult to treat. This is because as your body's master control system, the brain is critical to overall function (movement, speaking). Yet, the thick, bony skull that snugly protects this vital organ provides little room for the brain to swell.

Peterborough hospital was my first stop, but in realising the importance of complex surgery they had sent me off in one of the many ambulances on our roads to Cambridge.

Not much has been spoken of what must have been a heart-wrenching time full of doubt, despair and disbelief. I do know, however, that the three most important people in my life, the people feeling the most pain, at an early stage were told if I did wake I would be in a vegetative state and institutionalised.

A persistent vegetative state is a disorder of consciousness in which patients with severe brain damage are in a state of partial arousal rather than true awareness. It is a diagnosis of some uncertainty in that it deals with a syndrome. After four weeks in a vegetative state (VS), the patient is classified as in a persistent vegetative state. This diagnosis is classified as a permanent vegetative state (PVS) after approximately one year of being in a vegetative state.

I must quickly extinguish any negative path you may have taken during this particular quote and offer you comfort in the amount of progress that has been made to enable me to write this account.

All of this information was added much later. I was unconscious and completely unaware. When I say completely I suppose one would have missed an out of body experience, a light at the end of the tunnel, from what I gather there were a few near misses, so if there is a light I would have been able to see a flicker surely!

Roughly 5 percent of the general population and 10 percent of cardiac-arrest victims report near-death experiences, yet no one really knows what they are.

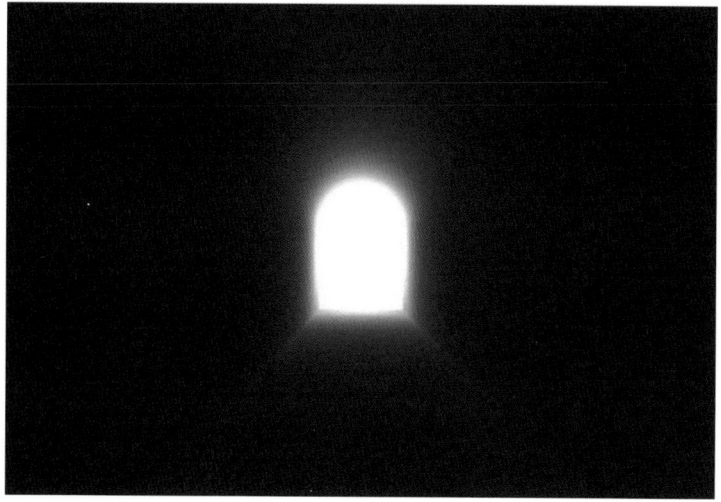

Example:

On a mountaintop looking out over a vast valley, with the wind blowing. I can feel it now whipping my hair about, and smell the clean smell of it. I hear the voices coming up to me, drifting up from the valley floor, telling me things. I feel the presence of a warm body behind me, holding me, so I rested comfortably to hear the voices of the wind.

"Who is to say I did not shake hands with God?"

Anyway, we will stick to my experience and try not to fantasise, that would be too easy considering the subject. Researching can only inform you of the facts, there is a lot left unknown about the issues experienced on this journey, and these may never be known.

Chapter 3

Recovery

Improvement, return to health, healing, revival.

Once I was stable, I was moved back to Peterborough Hospital into Rehabilitation, and my condition observed. This is where I awoke and was first aware of my surroundings. In a thick cloud trembling on the edge of consciousness the coming weeks would be hazy, nothing would make sense for days.

"My head was like an empty box lined with mirrors with a small hole. A beam of neon light in a suggestion, thought or question would enter. It shoots around, every surface hitting understood, every answer making complete sense until it finds the gap again. No sooner had it entered it disappears without any trace or trail of though left behind."

Not even forgotten, how can you forget if you never thought?

Consciousness refers to both wakefulness and awareness. Wakefulness is the ability to open your eyes and have basic reflexes such as coughing, swallowing and sucking. Awareness is associated with more complex thoughts and actions, such as following instructions, remembering, planning and communicating.

These are the skills I lost, was made to re-learn or adapt in the least disruptive way. I did not worry about talking or walking again, but I must have been more aware then. The room was getting smaller, details starting to make sense, every object fitted with some meaning or purpose. Until this point family and friends were coming and going without leaving much neon light in my box. The whole world was getting smaller rather fast.

Somewhere between dreams and consciousness I pulled out my catheter! Can you imagine the pain? A pain that finds the space between any words you might use to describe it, ducking and diving over and under all descriptive words associated with the rush of blood to your private area, ouch!

I had made a friend in the figure across the ward. I had been moved into the ward from a separate room to encourage my reactions and I suppose any social skills that may have been damaged. This not only enabled me to slowly become more aware, but also I could be observed by doctors and nurses to make sure my progress kept improving. My right arm in a very tight position was suffering from 'spasticity', which occurs in many similar cases. I believe it was treated with more then one injection of Botox.

I was communicating with shadows as they passed. Cheekiness, I'm glad to say was fully functioning, the nurses were subject to much of my inappropriate behaviour. The gap of a month or more I am afraid is lost in my library of memories, but I was making new ones every day from then on. I was seeing things in a certain light; I suppose the kind of light newborn babies see when they open their eyes upon the unknown.

Friends and family took me for walks around the ward and indeed the hospital in my wheelchair. I must make it perfectly clear, at no point was I trying to understand anything. After all my eyes had been seeing for twenty years, so there was not the questioning of the newborn, but more a kind of acceptance of the situation.

They had placed me under what is now known as the *Mental Capacity Act 2005*. Its primary purpose is to provide a legal framework for acting and making decisions on behalf of adults who lack the capacity to make particular decisions for themselves.

This means that while I lacked some mental capacity doctors and nurses made most of my decisions for me, from choice of clothes (a large selection of blue pyjamas), to what time I would get up and go to bed. All of this felt strangely comforting, leaving nurses to help you with everything we take for granted.

After several weeks of experiencing nothing, we sat in the hospital café so that my tired family could eat. Of course I'm only allowed tube food, but I can join in can't I? Everyone's being nice, as you would expect. Chatting and making pleasantries, my eye has not drifted from an open pack of Starburst sweets. Whoosh! I have snatched a Starburst, unwrapped it and popped it into my mouth quicker then you can say, "Tube food". It was the taste I expected! However, the two sets of hands down my throat were a tad un-comfy to say the least.

.

"It was a normal action, I could not think!"

To me it was a quick snap of time such as when you pick up the TV remote or some other unconscious movement to retrieve an object, food or otherwise. Shrouds of cover casting a shadow over my reality!

The family informed me later of the painstaking 3+ minutes it took to retrieve the sweet at a snail like speed that to me was the epitome of normal, but to the outside world was classic Brain Damage!

My brain had been put into slow motion, perhaps giving it time to recover where stem cells would have been reaching out to find comfort in connecting with others, at least finding an area to attach that left little distress.

Wheelchair bound I was looking in from the street outside. I think they thought it would 'widen my horizons', if only they had known how spacious and empty my life had been for the past couple of weeks. "Hey, hey!", What am I thinking I can't speak, Lord knows why?

An old college mate from my Stamford days hobbled by on crutches. Looking at me as if to say,
"Well?"
"Lets exchange stories".

I was pushed on. Although I could recognize his face as being familiar, the ability or desire was not there to talk or be stopped. Never forget the emptiness and acceptance of my current state of mind. The moment passed in seconds, but the trail of neon light lingered.

How does intention to speak become the action of speaking? It involves the generation of a pre-verbal message that is tailored to the requirements of a particular language, and through a series of steps, the message is transformed into a linear sequence of speech sounds. These steps include retrieving different kinds of information from memory and combining them into larger structures, a process called unification. Despite general agreement about the steps that connect intention to articulation, there is no consensus about their temporal profile or the role of feedback from later steps.

In addition, since the discovery by the French physician Pierre Paul Broca (in 1865) of the role of the left inferior frontal cortex in speaking, relatively little progress has been made in understanding the neural infrastructure that supports speech production.

I am aware of having a memory, being asked to draw in a square the layout of my bedroom as a kind of memory exercise. I am only just aware, as like many thick leather-bound novels there are no pictures. Just had an eerie sense of what has been.

Drew a perfect picture defining where my bed was, where my drawers were, where a keyboard on a stand stood, proud of my ability to retrieve such accurate information that seemed so urgent and important. It took a few seconds after being surprised at how quickly I was improving - my family sat startled! To take information from my damaged brain and transfer it onto paper took both concentration and memory!

"That's our last house", somebody said!
I was so confident and then one sentence threw everything into doubt. "Do you know where you are"?
My reply was, 'Denmark Hill'.

Those of you who know London will possibly know Kings College Hospital, where I spent some time about eight years earlier. It sits near the top of the hill and was my home for Euro 96, with Gareth Southgate stealing the show.

"Who is the Prime Minister?"

"John Major", I said confidently.

In the days of Tony Blair?

Although many other people were left dazed under Blair

It seems my brain had stepped over the messy pile of memories that had been scattered in a random pattern, and selected from the top of the neatly stacked memories just behind.

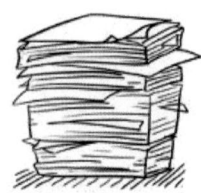

Chapter 4
Rehabilitation

Reintegrate, retrain, restore to health, readapt!

Rehabilitation is an active process, a series of steps to help people realise their optimal physical, mental, social and emotional potential; the steps for a stroke victim are slow and slight not always leaving an ideal outcome.

Modern research has shown that neuroplasticity is happening. Neuroplasticity (also known as cortical re-mapping) refers to the ability of the human brain to change as a result of one's experience, that the brain is 'plastic' and 'malleable', that the brain's cells' circuitry and interconnections can improve and strengthen with training and experience.

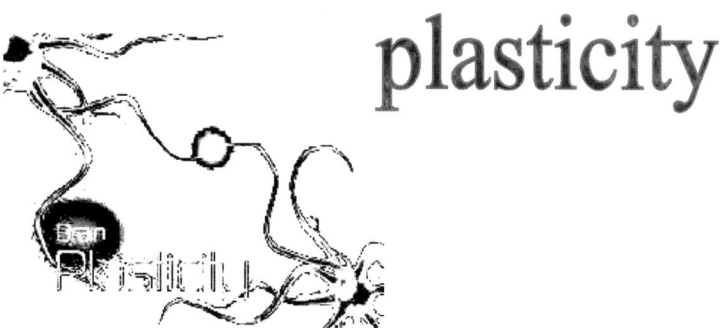

Neurosurgery is any kind of surgery used to treat a problem with the nervous system (the brain, spinal cord and nerves). In cases of severe head injury, neurosurgery is usually carried out on the brain. Neurosurgery is required in 1-3% of people with a severe head injury.

Every year in the UK, it is estimated that just less than 4,000 people have neurosurgery following a head injury. Possible reasons for neurosurgery include a haemorrhage (severe bleeding) inside your head, which puts pressure on the brain and may result in brain injury and, in severe cases, death.

Traumatic Brain Injury (TBI) is an Acquired Brain Injury (ABI) caused by a blow to the head or by the head being forced to move rapidly forward or backward, usually with some loss of consciousness.

Closed head injury is the most common cause of brain injury. It occurs when the head is struck or moved violently but the skull and/ or membrane lining of the brain is not broken or penetrated. Such damage often involves "diffuse brain injury" via widespread shearing, twisting and stretching of nerve fibres and bleeding due to the tearing of arteries and veins throughout the brain.

The forward motion and rotation of the brain on the relatively fixed brain stem is a common cause of loss of consciousness and coma.

An open head injury occurs when the skull and membrane lining of the brain have been fractured, cracked or broken so that the brain is exposed or penetrated. When an open head injury occurs, pieces of bone or cerebrospinal fluid may enter the brain. Considerable local damage can occur in the area immediately below the impact area, as well as more widespread damage.

My days would just be another section to be ticked off on a rehabilitation rota. I would have to rely on friends, family and, most importantly at this stage, the Nurses/HCAs who would feed, clothe and toilet me on a daily basis.

We would start the day by touching my nose for obvious reasons of assessing my coordination, eyesight etc. moving my way through what must have been a huge programme of therapy to walking un-aided.

As a result of this journey I was left with a debt of 99p, owed to an uncle who turned up at the right place at the right time.

Doctors had told my mother to try me on some soft food and while she was downstairs in the shop my uncle stopped by with an idle wallet. She returned to find me hiding behind a 99p cheeseburger, the best I ever tasted. I had not eaten solid food for weeks and was starving hungry! He would never let it drop. I paid him back!

My entire family would have to stay on their feet for a very long time to pay back the money spent on my recovery. With 24-hour care, machines running 24 hours a day, 24-hour on-call emergency first-aid, 24-hour Doctors, Nurses, Neurosurgeons, Physio- and Speech Therapists, Chefs, Porters, Cleaners and Laundry. All that was missing was a line of singing and dancing chorus girls!

The NHS came to my rescue like a shiny knight on horseback, waving his sword of death or glory, being fearless in the eyes of possible defeat, not to be outdone by any medical challenge or consideration of COST!

It was just the end of another day. I started wheeling myself out into the stairwell of Peterborough City Hospital - top floor. I think I was exercising my independence, showing nurses there was still activity upstairs, no matter how fleeting.

Then they began. Must have been 20 displays across the view I had. FIREWORKS! Magical at the time, but anybody will tell you it is the company that really counts. Without a feeling of sadness, or any feeling for that matter, I headed back to the Stroke Unit to engage in some mischief.

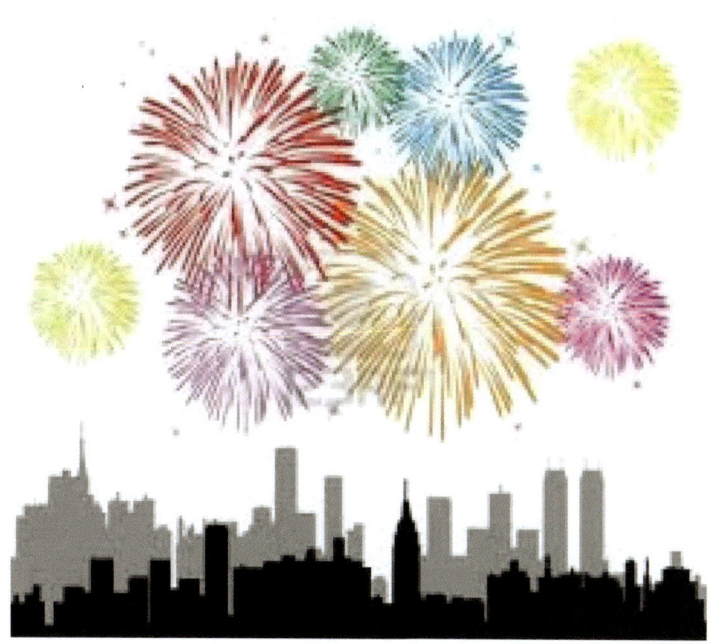

The Stroke Unit

This was my home for my stay in Peterborough. Although I had not had a stroke, I was left with similar impairments. I had spun my car one hundred and eighty degrees, slamming the driver's side into the only obstacle for yards – a large tree. I hit my head hard sending the energy shock surging down the right side of my body, leaving it incapable of performing even the most simple of tasks, and needing doctors with a needle to stimulate some kind of response.

The conditions were, I am told, wet. With the 'Renault Clio RT' facing the wrong way I was cut from it unconscious and bleeding. Some years later, I took a trip down to my local garage where a few of the retained firemen who did the cutting worked. I felt good knowing I was going to see and thank them. I think it must have been their day off!
So I convinced myself they would not like to see every life they had saved…

It shows how ironic life can be when it was my General Practitioner's wife on her bike who found me at the scene of the accident!

Without breaking a single bone I had sustained an injury which left me with a blood clot on the right hemisphere of the brain leaving me with Ipsilateral paralysis down the right side of my body.

Ipsilateral, (the same side).

This goes against common understanding, as the left hemisphere controls and receives information from the right side of the body and the right hemisphere controls and receives information from the left side.

Contralateral, (opposing sides).

Speech is usually controlled in the left hemisphere. Vision takes the combined effort of both hemispheres although the right hemisphere receives information from the left visual field while the left hemisphere receives information from the right. I have been trapped behind two rectangles of glass since 2003, sometimes with glare, sometimes without.

The right hemisphere (the one I damaged), dominates for perception, spatial ability, musical and artistic abilities, imagery and dreaming. The right hemisphere also seems to be more emotional and negative compared to the positive and rational left hemisphere. My punctured and deflated lungs were minor in comparison.

The surgeons removed a section of skull, which left the hole I referred to earlier. Need to get that filled if ever I am to hold on to thoughts let alone memories. Very important!

Recently I was reminded of layer upon layer of foot skin, ever so gently peeled back, like cigarette papers to a chain smoker endlessly whipping out his tin and handling the thinnest of Rizla with ease, even with hard, smoke-stained fingers, so confidently and firmly.

I was given a pumice stone, but with a mind scrabbling for thoughts and with one arm poised and ready to make some meaningful movements I started to uncover a foot, I am sure gasping for air.

The image in your head does not do it justice, it felt more like wax, pulling lumps out at a time leaving a gaping hole you could lose a toe in, occasionally drawing blood, but not enough to force me to stop.

You know when you're compelled to perform a task however long it takes, however fast it needs to be done, or however much pain is involved? I have realised that my brain damage pushes me through tasks with or without a blindfold. It gives me endless strength to complete them, while being very selective in those it chooses to undertake.

Sometimes I do forget to,

-BREATHE-

Addenbrooks my Graceland

In tough times you held my hand

Like a knight of the realm you came

Things would never be the same

Lost in thought

What a nice place to be

The wonderful feeling

Being free

A new life we shall see

The old lived so differently

Time lost

Time gained

Time to live again

Chapter 5
Coming home

I came home, as you do after a near fatal accident, to a newly painted bedroom with new wood furnishings. On the walls were hand painted designs in my favourite colour, green.

I cannot remember much about the transition between hospital and home, maybe because my box had not been sealed and memories were still escaping.

Nothing was being held on to, like a spaceman strapped into a spacesuit floating in a dark abyss with very little control over direction, taking away with him only pictures of stars and darkness or freewheeling down a hill on your bike and feeling the rush of danger and accomplishment. Pulling a skid one hundred and eighty degrees at the bottom, throwing dirt up into the air in a circle, like a stage-coach out of a Western and your mother clipping your lughole for putting her through such worry!!

Paralysis down the right side of my body, even loss of taste on the right side of my tongue, affected my coordination, so I could forget any kind of rhythm. Many scholars hold the opinion that it would almost certainly have returned to normal, but in so doing I would have had to endure years of 'practice guitar'.

As you guitar players will know, they are the worst years to be alive and I had a second chance, another go. I was not going to focus on my weaknesses, but my strengths. All I had to do was find them, re-focus my creative energy in the direction of an old Zimmermann (piano), left to me by my beloved Nana and Granddad.

I struggle to hold a rhythm in my strumming arm. It is easily done with the left hand on the piano, normally drowning out a badly held tune with my weaker right hand. Like many fine actors my left hand, arm and leg have taken the lead role in the film, 'Life of' leaving my right side to take the supporting role, a very important role to make the show a hit. I would be lost without the remaining function in my right arm but I let the left side lead.

The first map of the brain I looked at shows 'understanding humour' and 'move rhythmically' in the area where my brain was damaged. I hope when this is read you choose the same one I did, although I struggle to remember jokes!

Being pampered was very nice, and it lasted for months. Cortical re-mapping was taking place; stem cells were growing in places they had never grown before!
Changed personality?

"I will have to think about that!"

By the time I was home and had settled into a new kind of life, able to use the toilet without asking, able to make myself a drink and use a glass, able to step outside and walk (not too far), I was fully aware of the hole in my head, which of course was still there. I would ask people to touch my brain! What was even better was asking someone to run his or her hands through my hair. Of course I had to know them as they would inevitably leap back in horror asking,

"What is that?" as if I had lice!

Forget freewheeling! I had learnt a lesson from my second first-attempt at riding a bike.

"Like riding a bike", they say don't they?

I am confident, able to ride the street like Tyler Hamilton back then or Bradley Wiggins now. All was well until my core strength failed and I came down like a ton-of-bricks. I would have to adjust everyday life to my new capabilities. All could possibly improve, but for now I would have to adapt basic life skills.

We took a trip back to Addenbrooke's where my life was saved by a skilful neurosurgeon who, in my opinion is under-paid! Purpose you ask?

To, Replace and Retrieve. Replace the piece of skull they had removed and Retrieve the bit they took out, after all it was mine. Yes, yes! It is definitely mine. On asking a doctor for it, I was told,

"Sorry, it's not ours to give away"

"NO, ITS MINE!" I exclaimed.

Apparently as soon as any body part is taken out of your body it becomes the property of the taxpayer!

How dare he refuse my birthright, how very dare he?

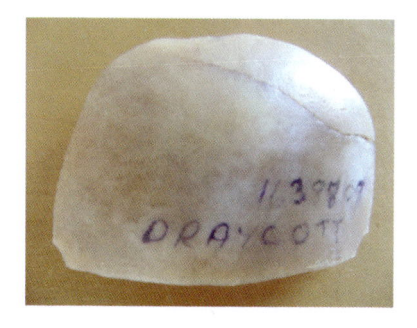

Section of skull

Ah, wait, I am getting ahead of myself.

Let me fill the gap.

(Excuse the pun)

Chapter 6

craniotomy

A craniotomy is a type of surgery that involves making a hole in your skull (the little reflective box) so that the surgeon can access your brain. This will be carried out under general anaesthetic so that you are unconscious and cannot feel anything. Once surgeons have accessed your brain, they will remove any blood clots that may have formed and repair damaged blood vessels.

Once bleeding inside your brain has stopped, the piece of skull can be re-attached or replaced. For me the chosen material was acrylic, not metal which is too heavy for the head. I had trouble on my feet as it was!

It was not the same bed I had used before, there was no life support machine, no ventilator, no tired nurse sat at the end of it and whatever else they needed to stabilise my life.

Once again I find myself waking to the sound of voices, this time warm friendly human voices, nothing standing out but mellow calmness. Lying down on my left side felt right. I was fully aware of the tube of blood from my head down to a bag acting as a drain.

My head felt sensitive, I did not dare touch and yet I could picture it looking horrific with a scar 32 staples long in a horseshoe design. It's for this reason lying on my left side is preferable to this day.

I do find comfort in the sound of surrounding human voices, letting me know the world is going about its business although I am taking a break. I had been in the world only hours earlier; there were no questions to be answered. I was told of the procedures, I am not sure how much detail was spoken of, but I knew.

You must have heard the term, 'Air Head'. When it is spoken the phrase is dismissed straight away with the knowledge that this could surely end a life.

Possibly the last thing you would like to hear from a Doctor after open head surgery is that the CT scan shows a fragment of trapped air! The safest place for air in the body is the lungs we all know this. Very common, we were told.

If it is that common why did I not know about it? A crash course in the, 'may never happens', would be both inappropriate and time consuming.

Best left to there and then.

After a day I was left with a panda's face. Two of the blackest eyes you will ever see. We are talking ten rounds with Tyson - black with swelling to match.

The most frustrating part of the black eye experience, apart from itchiness, is the lack of vision due to inflammation - another sense taken away temporarily, with thousands of blood cells going to work like a rich tomato purée on the boil. There was heat, my temperature rose like one of Mary Berry's English Muffins.

The black eyes went down as black eyes do and my days continued with a steady pace of re-learning and adapting the basics. Speech- and physiotherapy were administered over the following months. Considering the state I was in, they exceeded themselves. The professionals can only help guide you in the right direction.

"There are no wands to be waved in life"

Unfortunately, it comes down to hard work and persistence. I will be left with the changes to my body for the rest of my life. I would like to explain a few minor but very important impairments.

My right side feels the cold first and I lose some of the function in my right hand, arm, leg and foot, as if the accident was yesterday. When I focus on a detailed task, such as playing snooker, my right arm still sometimes makes involuntary movements that may cost me the game.

The speech patterns are obvious. It has taken years to accept in my head and not always practised,

"SLOW DOWN!"

Angry/frustrated/annoyed/impatient

The impairment that has changed my ability to walk the most is defined by the term, Roll *Slap*, Roll *Slap*. The sound of me walking on wood flooring, but I could feel it on any surface.

Our brain sends out many thousands of tiny electrical signals, which tell our bodies what to do. So when the brain is injured, there may be difficulties with movement. My right side was tight and right calf suffered from contracture (shortening of the muscle). While the left foot was hitting the floor, heel, toe, my right was just slapping. It's for this reason I could not walk at first, nor run, nor hop. Dorsiflexion - toe up to Plantarflexion - toe down.

Exercise:

Stand up, both feet heel and toe on the ground. Now hop without lifting onto your toe. See how much harder it is! Then try walking with flat feet.

I found not walking more frustrating than not speaking, the reason being, during my silent period I was not able to hold on to a thought for more than five minutes. I can only imagine living my life, dealing with the thousands of tasks we complete each day, in complete silence.

I have been speaking now for 9 years and 11 months, but I am still left with the impairment to my right leg, probably until I die.

"People take walking, talking, seeing, thinking, feeling and being for granted. I cannot explain how it feels to have all your human rights taken away so suddenly"

The brain minimises overload by balancing thoughts, memories and current affairs. Too much stress can cause anxiety which may result in the brain becoming exhausted, an 'unhealthy state of mind'. However, some stress and anxiety in moderation is, I believe, good for the mind as it quickens our powers of reasoning, positive thinking and problem solving.

To rest my brain I 'zone-out' from everything around me, slipping into a trance, letting all thoughts flash past like a slideshow running at speed, not stopping at any point to analyse or process them.

Positivity is a powerful healer. You see this in its active form every Saturday watching your football team. If they play well they will have been driven by positivity and confidence. At church, Pastors preaching with overwhelming positivity may work crowds up into such an ecstatic state that wonderful things happen - made happen by the creator, if you include evolution in the formula!

The possible effects of 'brain damage' are clearly outlined in documents available in all medical facilities. They include feeling anxious, less sociable, irritable, which may lead to changes in the way you think or communicate with others, and in the way you manage everyday tasks. Physiological effects can include difficulty with walking, including balance and coordination. I am often saying hello to doorframes.

Migraines are a relatively new unwanted effect in my life. Nine times out of ten the relief when they end is accompanied by a vomiting episode. Not pleasant!

The migraine was a monster, a head throbbing evil worm in my control system hacking into my sight making the eyes feel heavy, like when you stare at an Hawaiian shirt for too long, seeming to make your retinas bleed while twitching his toes that are grounded in your stomach making you as sick as a dog. Then hanging around through paracetamol doses, water attacks and as much calmness as you can throw at it. Once vomited, it decides it has had enough fun and leaves without any trace.

Can you remember the figure across the ward - my friend? We spent a lot of nights roaming the halls of Peterborough city hospital together, on the same wavelength, understanding each other, although looking back we were two very confused people. I always got the feeling he was looking out for me, taking me under his wing as an experienced stroke victim. It was not his first, and he was not a day over 35.

We had exchanged numbers only for me to learn he had died…

R.I.P
Paul

Chapter 7
Back to the Grindstone

My placement in the sweet factory was different. I had previously been in the boiler room, folding the hot sweet mix and rolling it into a huge sausage roll, spreading any necessary toffee or jam, then lifting it into the machine that sends it though a die to cut out the Rosy Apples or Aniseed Twists. No more!

Packing was better suited for someone with 'brain damage'. Pouring the box of fresh smelling newly cut sweets into another machine that individually wraps the little hard boiled, sticky when sucked, lumps of sugar!

My healing mind was taking control of life like never before. I was growing up and things had to change. Legs were walking, head was thinking, mouth was speaking and I had a life that needed living.

I cannot remember any particular difficulties because my brain had accepted my new abilities quicker than my body. So if a task was beyond me it was simply a case of it being too hard and not connected to the injury itself.

There is no way I could have completed any of the tasks in my last position in the factory, but then there are millions of people who never have.

It is all a question of perspective and being thankful for our current capabilities. There will always be someone stronger and smarter than you, which only emphasises the letter 'I', the one not found in the most valuable lesson taught at the earliest of ages: **T.E.A.M.**

We were working as a solid unit, a team of people selling to countries as far away as America. This was a well-oiled, mechanical process of pumping glucose into the boiler room, after which it spent the day with us being transformed before boxing-up to be sent out when ordered by an overweight population, thereby keeping dentists on their toes and contributing to the bad habits we have all embraced.

There are lots of wrongs in the world like foreign drivers or red cards; trouble is many of them are out of our hands. Right any wrongs you see and are able to, or head to the bathroom and start washing your hands in public.

Hindsight would be an earth-changing discovery, just think of all the wrongs that could have been right!

I had spent every evening for three long years during this re-placement to become a qualified Graphic Designer - my original goal, my destination if you will.

This was the chosen path for me, chosen by my keen eye for detail, not forgetting my 'A' in art at school.

"Ones creative hands"

I come from a creative family; why not follow the path laid out for me by the laws of genealogy. The ABI has pushed me out of the family line and, like 'Back-To-The-Future 2', on 1st August 2003 my timeline skewed off to run an alternative life.

Although I still carry the genes, I no longer possess the steady hand or vision that was passed on to fulfil my original potential. The gene may be passed on, but for me it will have to be re-learnt, adapted or lost forever.

Life goes on and risk continues to be a part of it. In fact it was an accident, a consequence that shows how vulnerable humans are when, tiredness, laziness and distraction combine to become a determining force!

Most people chuckle to themselves when they see a sign saying, 'Tiredness Kills, Take Breaks'. I have since slept in petrol stations. Taken too far? Maybe, but I am here to tell you about it which is a gift to me and anybody else who can remember a time of nothingness.

They are called accidents, as there is a percentage chance of you not having one. You should never rely on chance!

"The chance of me not having an accident today is good!"

Thought is a powerful tool, do as much thinking as you can. Try never to regret your thoughts, only learn to think more! Weigh-up risks, danger and I plead with you to consider the weather when driving!

You know how people see things in you that you couldn't believe, for you thought the complete opposite. Well somebody saw something in the new if damaged me and made this life changing comment,

"Ever tried caring?"

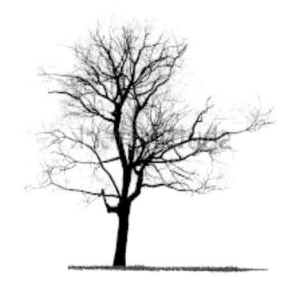

Chapter 8
A New Hope

I got the job without much effort. It was something new, something to get me away from the past. Little did I know that years later I would be saying in interviews that it was the best introduction to caring I could have had. The reason for this was the wonderful characters I cared for whilst employed there.

- Bipolar
- Down's syndrome
- Epilepsy
- Prader-willi
- Autism

I was set up for a career in the caring community with work training that would improve my movements, actions and speech patterns in a work environment. The hard reality is it was all re-programming my own brain for a life that had been so suddenly saved.

The things I saw were shocking, until I became used to the behaviour. This happened very quickly. Being thrown in at the deep end is an understatement. Within the first year I was completing daily logs and risk assessing through to administrating medicines, filling out the relevant paper work and MAR Charts (Medicine Administration Record).

I had acquired my level 2 NVQ (National Vocational Qualification), in Health and Social Care. The awarding body for this was Oxford Cambridge and RSA Examinations (OCR), and the regulatory authority was the Qualifications and Curriculum Authority (QCA). I also pulled in NCFE Level 2 in Safe Handling of Medicines and Level 2 Award in Food Safety and Catering.

An NVQ Qualification is a qualification that assesses someone's competence (that is the skills, knowledge and understanding they have), principally in a work situation.

It is about direct care, where the focus is hands-on care, enablement care, development and maintenance of the client's independence and helping patients, clients or service users to boost independence and encourage their minds to think positively.

The list of work based evidence to prove you have met the requirements for an NVQ is as follows;

- Your practice/performance
- Your reflective accounts
- Case studies
- Products of your own work and contributions you have made, such as care plans, minutes, reports, project reports, etc.
- Witness testimony
- Service user testimony
- Answers to oral and written questions
- Written assignments and projects
- Previous experience and learning

All of this practice in reading, writing and speaking would help my mind adjust/re-adapt to my new abilities. I would strongly advise any victims of brain damage to enrol on a work-based course of some description, where you are given a clear goal to aim for. The Open University runs a range of free courses including, 'Starting with Psychology'.

Imagine a self-acclaimed 'cool dude' stood in a living area observing patients. In walks an autistic man. Down go his trousers like a primary school boy. With pants and joggers round his ankles, and before I could believe what my eyes were seeing, he started urinating. I must have thought of a hundred reactions, but before I could decide on any of them, the carpet had a small puddle and he was still peeing!

A story that might demonstrate how one brain-damaged individual could empathise with another began on Halloween night in my first year.

We were at a party. There was music, and a few uncomfortable staff. Sufferers of bi-polar disorder can experience behavioural extremes and one man so afflicted suddenly became very anxious. Study suggests bipolar disorder may cause progressive brain damage. While everybody ran away he stood with a slightly confused look on his face wielding a large picnic bench above his head. Breathe! I watched him throw the bench, approached him, and sat with him until he was calm. Days later my manager decided to call me into the office and praise me. Had I done something out of character?

The Latin phrase, cogito ergo sum,

"I think, therefore I am", is a philosophical proposition by René Descartes. The simple meaning is that thinking about one's existence proves - in and of itself - that, an "I" exists to do the thinking. This proposition became a fundamental element of Western philosophy, as it was perceived to form a foundation for all knowledge. While other knowledge could be a figment of imagination, deception or mistake, the very act of doubting one's own existence arguably serves as proof of the reality of one's own existence, or at least of one's thoughts.

For many people who suffer from brain injury, the problems associated with it become a permanent part of their lives. The problems that develop depend upon which part of the brain is injured. The most unnerving consequence of a brain injury can be,

A change in personality!

The function of a specific area of the brain is a defining characteristic of an individual's personality and when damaged it can appear as if a new person has taken their place. This is how I feel sometimes without any regret about the accident itself. Am I supposed to regret the day I started showing more empathy, compassion, understanding, and patience?

My taste in music has not changed, my taste in clothes has not changed, my taste in books - I have never been a reader! I had no idea where my career was going and was left confused with where it had been. I was definitely in the right place.

Everybody is an individual and receives fulfilment in different areas of life. I think I was starting to understand my confused personality. I was searching for visible signs of improvement in others and myself, this would happen over days, weeks, months and even years.

One day my phone rang. It was a friend from pre-crash days. They were ever so excited as they always were. They said, "You will never guess who is on my course?"

I had no idea that they had enrolled on a Mental Heath Nursing Course at - you guessed it - Addenbrooke's.

"Who?" I asked.

It turned out to be my cousin, who I had not seen for a long time. Funny, how I'd been steered in the same direction.

I would like to think it was because of my accident he chose this path, but I think it is just a case of chance. I am not spiritually driven in any way, shape or form. My views are based purely on observation and personal experience.

Staying with a good friend and cousin in the student accommodation, sneaking around the underground passageways eating crisps I seem to remember, and being within 100 kilometres of my 'Graceland' that gave me back a future, was very special.

I would like to take this opportunity to deeply thank the following Mental Health Nurses for their strong, binding and therapeutically healing friendship through this challenging time of self-discovery and rehabilitation.

David Draycott, Esther Linger, Helen Hughes, family and friends none of whom has ever turned their back on me, although acceptance can sometimes be tricky to fully achieve.

Thank You

We did go back to the room where I drew some life-saving breaths. Although my family knew their way around and stood reminiscing, I had no emotion, no memory of the place. I was walking around a Hospital - my family were walking around painful memories!

Never have I ever reacted to bad news more gracefully than the day all the staff members were asked to line up outside the managers office.

The tension was like a soft cheese on slate. To be cut!

People were entering the office then filing out of the side door never to be seen again. We were being laid off, made redundant! I dealt with the owner, who was performing the unpleasant duty, in a very appreciative way, trying to show my gratitude for the experience he had provided. I think it took him completely off guard.

I thanked him for the opportunity to try this new experience, shook him firmly by the hand, and walked out feeling like a **King!**

If you ever get the chance, try it.

Chapter 9

Educating the Anxious

Now this was a big step, I had gone from being a 'cool dude', to teaching autistic children. It sounds lovely, but the reality was a lot different.

You may as well stand me outside a nightclub in Brixton as a bouncer in a black suit, looking very smart and important, but ending up being beaten every day and night. But my new approach to situations was based on empathy, compassion and understanding, so in a way I was glad to be hit by an anxious child.

I was communicating, hopefully making a difference. But at the end of every day, sadly, in such a short space of time there were no visible signs of change and I suppose in that type of situation you can become weary and bruised. Don't get me wrong the experience was fantastic, I learnt a lot! The training in behaviour, communication and safeguarding would help me as I progressed through my journey.

Autistic people need a framework and depending on where they are on the autistic spectrum will determine how strict the routine is they will need to follow.

We would use many tailored techniques with the challenging behaviour that was displayed daily, putting into practice the training we were given which was updated quarterly.

P.R.O.A.C.T.S.K.I.P - (Positive Range of Options to Avoid Crisis and use Therapy Strategies for Crisis Intervention and Prevention).
T.E.A.C.H - (Treatment and Education for Autistic and Related Communication-Handicapped Children).

A positive approach would be used thereby focusing on what could be done rather than what could not.

When a client's care plan states that something has to be done in a particular way due to the condition, it can cause problems with the individual involved when they request all manor of duties, activities or tasks and you only have the one approach.

When carrying out risk assessments I would check existing ones to ensure there was no contradictory information/assessments to avoid creating difficult situations and maximise a 'low arousal' atmosphere.

Blank canvas or fresh start, breathe and re-focus. All suited me down to the ground, although I was unsure why at the time.

Families and authorities from all over England had rejected these particular children. There were highs and bruises, but I think my compassion and understanding of what it's like to be trapped inside your body and misunderstanding everything helped me give the best I have.

I will always remember going skateboarding with an autistic lad. He never spoke but seemed to understand things better than me at times. However, it was the same lad that took off the tip of my left index finger!
In the car, off the drive and into the street,
Who is that calling?

"Come back, we have your finger!"

Listen, I have nothing to moan about, for there is always luck hiding behind every grey curtain of misfortune. Each time a job comes to an end, I find myself a better placement. When I have crashed a car, they seem to reward me with a better one.

I had been taken to the best hospital after my ABI and when I lost my finger I had the best plastic surgeon working on hands in England to keep as much length as possible enabling me to continue playing the piano.

Many day and night shifts went by after my return.
I felt low and empty, a feeling I knew only too well.

Sometimes in those moments where you let you mind wander, plan, organise, skills I no longer take for granted, I try to fill the gap in time that has been lost. It hurts not to have memories on the border of teenage years and adulthood.

It is impossible to find memories from before and place them anywhere near the date of the accident. Like a void, this period is empty, blank, abyss, gulf, nullity, oblivion.

"The blank void of space"

I love this reference:

The Children's Trust

For children with brain injury.

Our memory works rather like a high-speed version of a huge library. New information comes in to our heads much as a new book arrives at a library. The memory has the job of processing it and giving it the right label before sending it to the appropriate section and shelf. A brain injury can make this system much less effective, and sometimes the information isn't always sent to the right place. Problems with memory occur when we go looking for something amongst the shelves, but it isn't in the section it's supposed to be. An injured brain has to work that much harder to find what it's looking for as it scours the whole of the library.

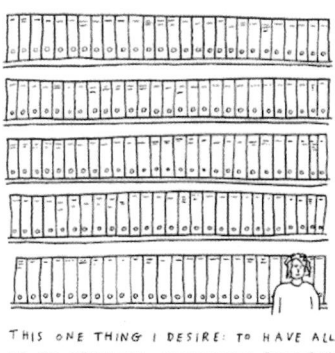

THIS ONE THING I DESIRE: TO HAVE ALL OF MY PERSONAL PAPERWORK SENSIBLY ARRANGED IN LABELLED BOX FILES

Stanford Encyclopedia:

*"Memory is one of the most important ways by which our histories animate our current actions and experiences. Most notably, the human ability to conjure up long-gone but specific episodes of our lives is both familiar and puzzling, and is a key aspect of **personal identity.** Memory seems to be a source of knowledge."*

.

I moved on again, to create more memories, looking for new challenges, something to enlarge my library of experience

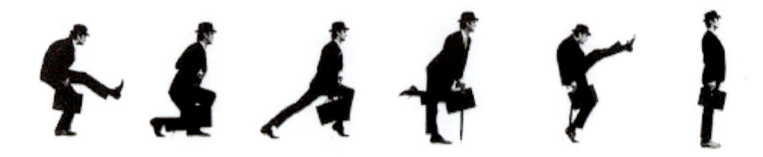

"Everyday is a lesson in human behaviour, mannerisms and being prepared for the unpredictable!"

Chapter 10
The Climb

Reaching the top was a life saving breath of fresh air pumped into the lungs, not by a ventilator, but by....

We started the idea with a trip to our local Army shop, (Home Guard Field Supplies), for the gear to tackle an endurance test, to see if I was nearing my normal ability. I was confident in mind, but I knew by then not to rely on thought alone!

After a beautiful drive we arrived at one of the many campsites. Tent packed and a bit thirsty, we stopped in a hiker's pub with drinks flowing, fire roaring and a small Dachshund called Colin.

When exchanging chat with the Welsh barman (as much as we could), we were told of a 'Lovely Little Cottage' nearby that they rented out to other inexperienced climbers.

We asked him how much and, weighing up price, landscape and weather - all being terrible - we opted out of the tent and into the Cottage. Sounds warm, comfy, rather luxurious one might say.

Given directions we pulled up outside a gorgeous, stone built, lockable box.

Honestly, there was not enough room to swing a cat, if you could get the cat in with you. But it was still preferable to a tent and it was beautiful, with a small river alongside. The 'Valley's' were our garden and we soaked up all the wonders of the wilderness with walks over streams, fences and through sheep poo!

The morning of the climb we awoke to a still-air atmosphere, Radio 1 on the wind-up radio and a hot cup of tea from the kettle on the stove provided. It was a lovely day, bursts of sunshine, but not overwhelmingly hot, after all we had left our sunscreen at home.
It was summertime but that does not apply in the 'Valley's'.

Key dropped off we started the pleasant walk through a couple of fields to find an appropriate track. Track found we start to zigzag through gates and fields with nothing but the opinion that this was a grand idea.

After about an hour things started to get a bit trickier than expected. The slope had become a touch steeper with more rocks! Another hour passed quite quickly, it was never going to be a minimal-effort stroll, the weather turning cloudy, which was to be expected, and the slope steeper. After all we were climbing a hill!

The light was being turned down as if controlled by God himself, and the clouds started raining, I am sure out of God's control. Wind was now cutting in, from the east?

The rain was coming down so hard, if I took off my hat I thought my head would bleed. I had no idea how far we had gone or how far we had to go. Eventually we were crouched down in the foetal position in fear of being blown off the hill.

At this point the reconstruction should have started being performed by two handsome actors wearing thick coats and shiny boots. No chance! If we'd had a signal, yes, it would be 999! However, looking back, a number for mountain rescue would have been more appropriate.

Between short breaks of rain we would continue up the mountain reaching what felt to be (could not see), a train track. Four of an estimated three hours passed; we were weary and had not eaten. The next forty-five minutes were almost as bad as 'practice guitar'.

I am forgetting to mention my right arm and leg, which were numb, probably because my brain has accepted the change to my body's ability, therefore, (to me), not as important as telling you about the weather. I can only apologise.

Reaching the top was a life saving breath of fresh air, pumped into the lungs, not by a ventilator, but by…

...the hot air fans just past the 'Star Trek' style doors that opened out of nowhere through curtains of thick mist. It was very dark by this point, cold, wet, with a wind to take your head off, but we had reached our goal that at the time was our 'Graceland'. Just past the 'Star Trek' doors, just past the hot air fans, stood four vending machines, and beyond them was a fully working open kitchen with tables, chairs and a gift shop where we were to purchase a certificate of our achievement – the climbing of Mount Snowden.

Surrounding all this was a pane of glass looking out from the top of the mountain as if they were expecting a sunny day? We sat warm, but wet-through, to a hot meal and drinks contemplating how to get down like we had popped to the local shop for milk!

Whoever made the decision to catch the train back down was doing so out of shame. Just as we sat down in briskly walked a class of school children shouting,
"Lets do it again",
Surely they meant the train ride?

We caught the 999 back down. Unfortunately it twists itself around to stop on the wrong side of the second largest mountain in UK, which left more walking to the car! Once more my feet were grounded in lead filled boots and my head was again out of the clouds.

The difficulties people with brain injuries face are easily ignored or misunderstood. Even family members and friends may regard a person with Acquired Brain Injury who exhibits cognitive problems or changed behaviour, as lazy or hard to get along with.

I have found my lack of expression or displayed emotion has irritated people. Imagine you're filling yourself with emotion, spilling your heart out - to a zombie!
Just because you are not displaying emotion doesn't mean you are not feeling. You must look somewhere else for your expected reaction, body language or behavioural patterns. Communication is a two-way channel. If person two is not on the same page, you're not communicating, it then becomes a speech. This is why the best reply to a heckle is not to react!

Chapter 11
Experienced

My induction training went well. I was experienced in behaviour, had worked with all ages with every learning disability I could name. I had seen everything that I wished to see.

I was posted lone-working with an autistic man who suffered with a condition called Polydipsia. Easier to work with than many, just a constant thirst - manageable!

Every day would focus on enhancing his independence and enabling him to live his life safely in the way he chose.

His behaviour was improving as witnessed by my manager and more importantly his family, who we would visit weekly.

We had built a strong bond using body language due to him being profoundly deaf. We were able to read each other's every next move through routine and our predictable likes/dislikes that made living with him three days and nights a week rewarding in very different ways.

He found his reward through feeling safe, comfortable and cared for. Mine was that warm feeling you get when you let somebody out at a junction or give someone your parking ticket.

I do believe that the very strict routines that I implemented in the residential schools were an important tool when adapted to his level of autism that was minor in comparison.

The role enabled me to help him in the way experience had shown me.

Work was living!

My day...

My name is _____

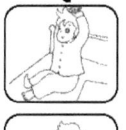

I get up at

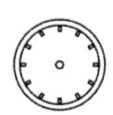

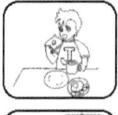

I eat breakfast at

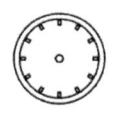

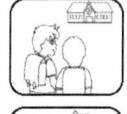

I go to school at

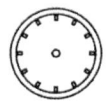

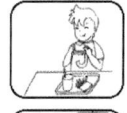

I eat lunch at

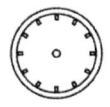

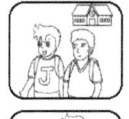

I leave school at

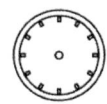

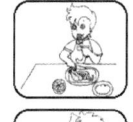

I eat dinner at

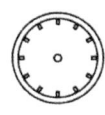

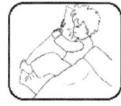

I go to bed at

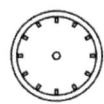

I find the human mind fascinating, unbelievable, a work of art. I have met many lovely characters thanks to the change in my circumstances and been part of some magical experiences, involving people with such varied abilities that I would never have understood before my accident. I find it difficult to imagine a life with no crash.

If you think back to a safely stacked, correctly labelled pile of books in your office upstairs, to when ponies could fly, He-Man was a hero and the ice cream van had always run out of ice cream, you will undoubtedly see that it was in fact a brain with time and space to explore the heights of imagination and the realms of reality, always choosing ponies or He-Man over your mother's instructions.

A description or visual expression of what brain damage is like would be when Jerry has hit Tom over the head with a frying pan. The combination of animated stars above his head and dazed expression on his face is a good way to portray to the viewer all they need to know about the consequence of Jerry's actions and Tom's feelings at the time.

This simplistic display is probably the most accurate, almost as if at some time in the past the animator has been through the same experience and come up with stars to express the emptiness.

Brain damage in me has once again created space. I do try to find the time to think outside my mirror lined box to fill the space, perhaps not of flying ponies or He-Man, but of things unimportant that make me happy.

"'The Humans' try so hard to live their life with meaning and purpose; they neglect the thoughts of HAPPINESS!"

"We don't have long. Be happy!"

Chapter 12
Trip of a Lifetime

I was asked one day if I wanted to go to Israel and grabbed at the chance with both hands.

We saw all the biblical sights I knew about thanks to my primary school education. But this was a university degree in sightseeing. Every story taught in the Bible was seen plus a dip in the Dead Sea, which contains 33% salt, too much for my eczema, but deemed to be healing and therapeutic. It was a while ago but 'hey' I'm game.

Now if you have never had a real culture shock, this is probably not the ideal place to be outside of an arranged-Christian-group, although you would be in the minority.

Never before had I felt so excluded, and that is saying something. Israelis are friendly enough, just a cultural barrier to be broken by any brave, confident, social superman.

AS A GROUP WE GO TO SEE THE GOLD STAR

WHERE PEOPLE CELEBRATE THE BIRTH

OF JESUS CHRIST

IN THE NATIVITY CHURCH BETHLEHEM

KNELT DOWN TO TOUCH THIS SACRED STAR

*I get the feeling we were looking
for Acknowledgement of our
Forever thankfulness*

~~thank you~~
~~hea's~~
~~bed~~
~~nurses~~
~~hospital~~
~~ambulance~~
~~first-aid~~
~~doctors~~

~~addenbrooks~~
~~a life saved~~
~~a new person born~~

-You need no words in such a moment-

Spending ten days understanding only the conversation within your small group was in a way frustrating – a rather familiar feeling of exclusion. Life is full of such feelings, and the person who discovers the power of choosing which feeling to feel will be, in more ways than one - Rich!

Understanding speech patterns is crucial to conversation, otherwise whole paragraphs can be taken completely out of context. In my case, it is especially my dry sarcasm I have had to keep an eye on. I have found myself offending people in an innocent sentence or joke about a slightly controversial subject.

And so I have landed, settled into my seat and sat back for the feature film, 'Life Of '. When I have a bad day and ones head is full of unwanted thoughts, I do try to remember life without a care in the world. It was much easier to let each day drift by, as opposed to living each day with meaning and, most importantly, purpose.

I have gone from no thought to wanting rid of thoughts and I hate myself for it. You should never regret thought, it is only action that can change the direction of events that may have needed more thought, not less!

Without an old personality to compare with, I feel I have been left with a new one in essay form to read through and start living by, surprising myself at some actions that were hidden in the small print at the back!

I have in fact been living my life for the past ten years inside a big bouncy bubble not to be deflated by any negative news that just ricochets off to land somewhere else.

I think this bubble was left due to trapped wind after open head surgery, leaving me with no choice but to live some sort of lie. Within this bubble I have been gazing out at stars and sunsets with an overwhelming sense of appreciation for the glorious images given to us in a random selection.

Brain damage has changed the way I emotionally respond to commonplace occurrences that test us daily. I have blended into the stomach of society slowly picking out the flaws in my character that separate me from the normal.

"A cascade of emotions, feelings and thoughts, falling into a pool of realisation using paddles of acceptance to wade through the treacherous waters"

I had not felt many feelings during the early days after my ABI, although my family I am sure were swamped in them. I try not to think of reactions. When I do, I break down. Through curiosity I have asked a few questions to which the answers were horrific! Not quite enough to make me a 'believer'! But I have thanked where thanks are due, to bring a sense of peace for my brain to process in it's own time.

This must be my deserved rest after the trauma of previous years. My head was now ready to move on.

"Where are we with no

Emotion, Feeling or Thought

Who can discover without a

Lesson Learnt

Would the world still turn with

Equal Passion

Or is it an individual journey of

Appreciation

The world spins with

Aptitude & kindness

So take a moment   −breath−

give your talent to those who need it

Explore the Heights

Explore the Lows

For the challenges we will encounter

No Body Knows"

I turned my attention to a unit back in Peterborough.

Sir Tony Robinson opened the building on the 9th September 2013, a neurological care unit just across the road from the new City Hospital.

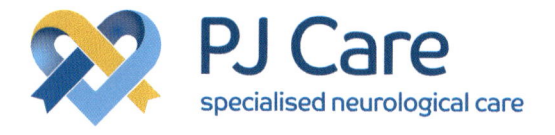

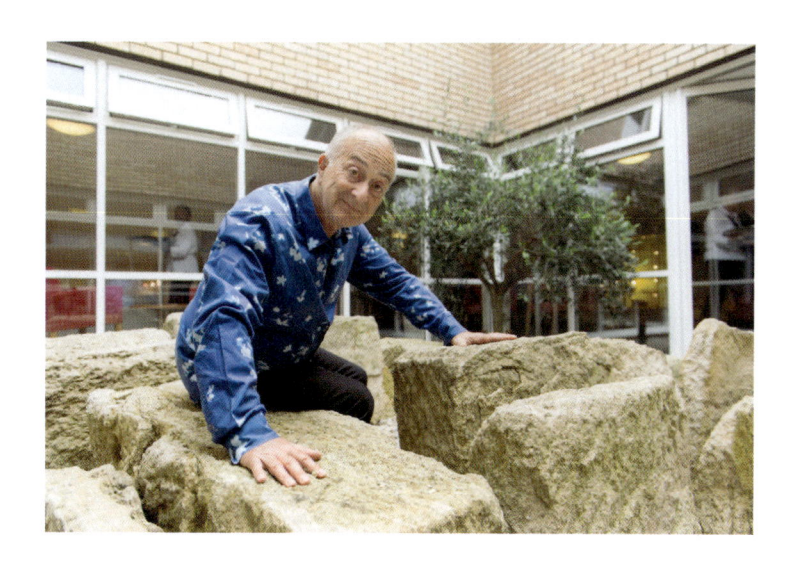

Chapter 13
2013 Self-Fulfilment

This would be something special, starting this journey with nothing more than a small collection of memories in a damaged mirror lined box, to helping the body's natural goal of rehabilitating itself in the many damaged control systems I would meet each day.

Could this be it, my destiny if such a thing can be found? I told them my skills would be best placed with learning disabilities!

"Neuro-Rehabilitation"

I said, with some sort of understanding of what to expect. That's where I want to be, making a difference, helping people with sustained neurological conditions and seeing them come in, opening their eyes upon the unknown and making sense of it - filling the emptiness.

Ten years after my crash, the news came through today.

I have been given the greatest pleasure in becoming a member of the Neuro-Rehabilitation Team!

2013

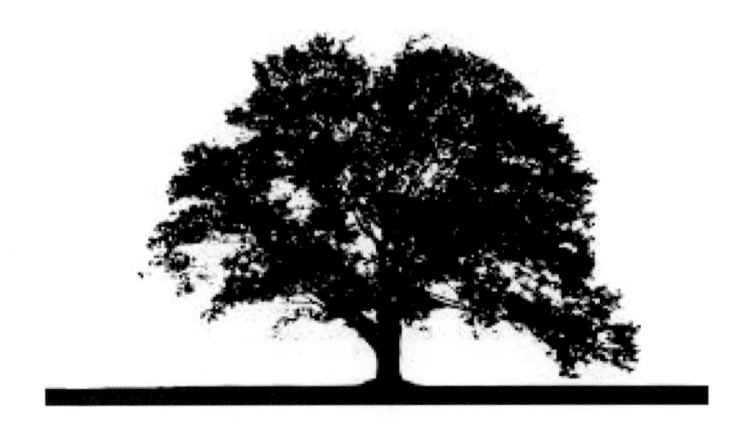

HCA: Neuro-Rehabilitation

Giving back to the world the care and
time it gave to me

Walking

Through the ward today

And seeing a 20-year-old lad with a scar on his head,

Was emotional. I don't know much about his situation,

But looking into his eyes I could see

Traces of thought inside

His – **Reflective** – **Small** – **Box**

A true story **2013**

REPLACED!

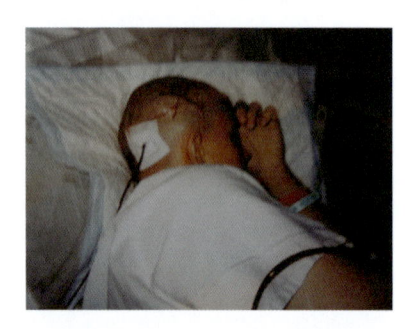

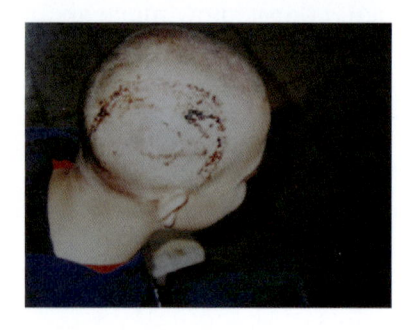

RETRIEVED!

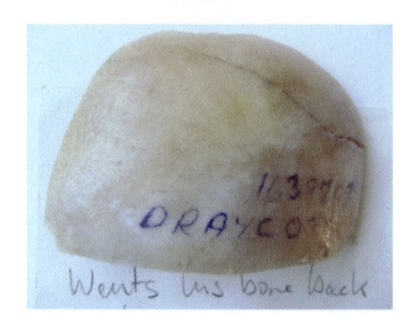

PJ Care
specialised neurological care

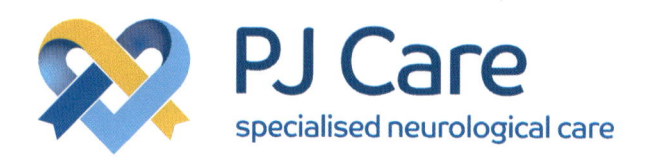

PJ Care is a leading provider of specialist neurological care and neuro-rehabilitation for people with progressive or acquired neurological conditions.

I was very impressed when entering to be greeted by an open reception area, glass-surrounding a Roman well, and so well presented.

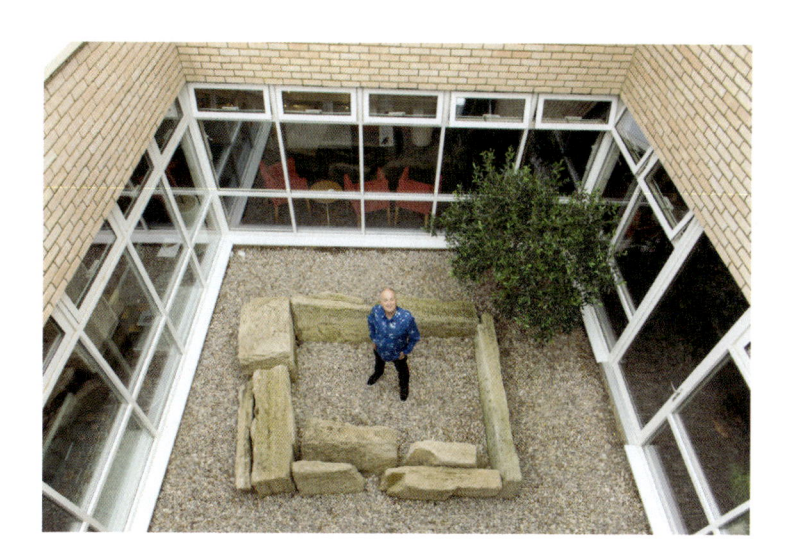

The place is shiny new, automatic doors, many floors and training rooms, high and low gardens, on site hydrotherapy pool, skills kitchen, therapy room and nursing stations.

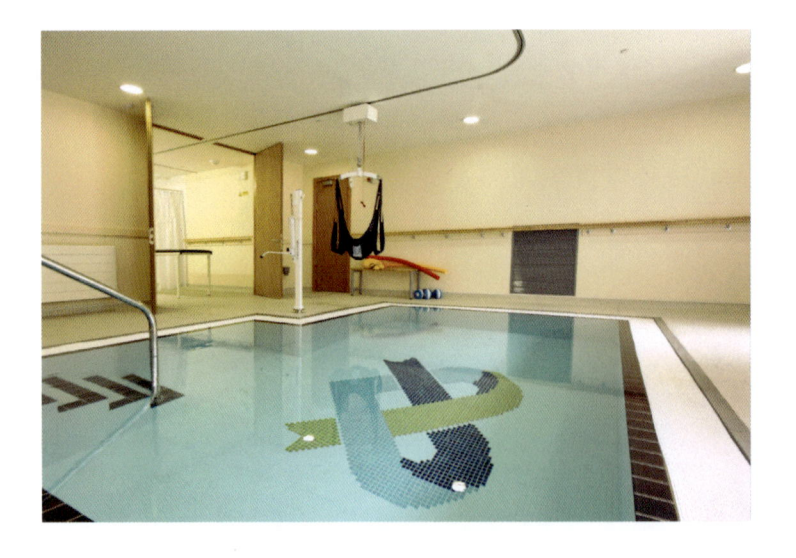

All this is very important, but without the dedicated staff giving away endless love it would feel empty.

Passing the Baton

If you had told me ten years ago that in 2013 I would have made a miraculous recovery and would be a trained Health Care Assistant (HCA) working in Rehabilitation, I would have found enough strength and breath to whisper, DREAMS.

At times it has been emotionally hard with many hurdles, but you should never give up on life, only learn to work alongside it and jump higher.

Almost settled in now and I have already made some contributions towards peoples' recovery, along with the special lad that almost brought me to tears. My future now is working alongside physiotherapists and nurses to encourage bruised minds and broken stem cells to find their optimal potential. Already I have found my psychological limits by wiping a man's brow, only to find his room empty the next day.

'The sudden realisation of life and its end!'

I have been actively assisting physiotherapists in the gym and hydrotherapy pool and in a short space of time picked up and dropped off patients. I have witnessed an endless progression of improvements in others.

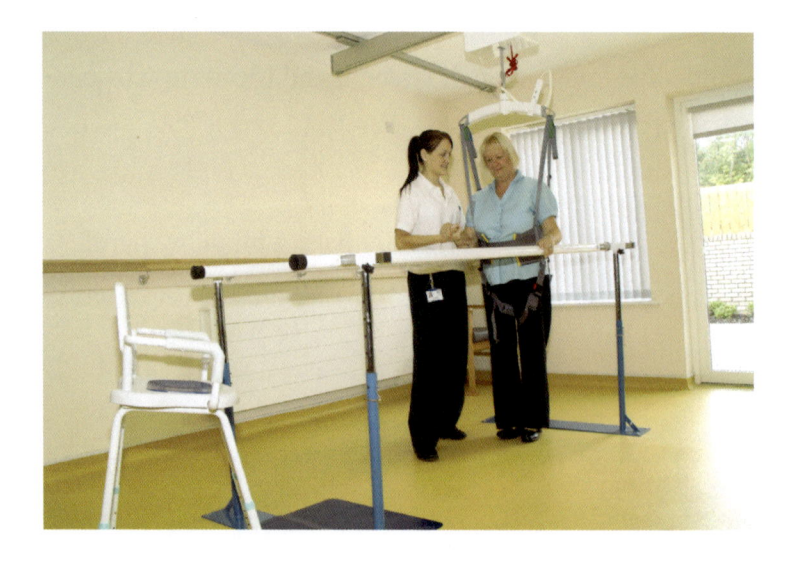

This is living!

We have all been playing a game called, 'Balloons' and I find myself continuously using my stronger arm while telling Curtis to use both hands!

It is very important to stimulate muscles that have had some kind of trauma, to recover as much movement as possible.

Everyday he is becoming more aware and with that comes the frustration, made worse by the fact he can't hold on to thought for more then a few moments, wondering what this empty space is and why he is in it!

Like a cassette on loop he keeps realizing his situation and it p****** him off!

One day I was required to accompany Curtis to hospital. As his hands were making some meaningful movements, he pulled out his Peg Feed from his stomach. Can you imagine the pain, I am not sure he could.

That was the last time he took medication via Peg, he was crying out for normality.

His journey will be unique, I wish him the best of luck, but it will take determination, motivation and an incentive to achieve a recovery he can be proud of.

With him being very smart, his brain is used to a lot of activity, so he scours his huge library for the answers he has to questions that are posed. This is positive thinking.

Minds must become hungry when damaged.

"I am starving hungry!"

Now this is due to one of two things, either the army of cells working over time, all the time, to complete an urgent repair job on the commanders head office, matching paint and carpet want a lunch break, or a lack of taste, feeling, satisfaction and energy.

A long awaited weekend arrives, where Curtis is off to - you guessed it - Addenbrookes, to replace a section of his box. I spend some of the proudest days of my life being able to offer support to another family who are living this nightmare.

I was staying in the student accommodation where I had slept before as a guest, but this time I was staying as a trained HCA. I felt very honoured walking the corridors of Addenbrooks in my uniform, wearing my ID badge with pride and smiling to myself knowing how lucky, privileged and fortunate I was to be staying there in those circumstances.

Memories flood back, hopefully suggesting the right words to comfort and support.

Distraction has been a useful tool when alleviating anxiety or pain. I tell a story of an experience only to be interrupted by his sister,

"Curtis has been though the same!"

We became closer with the closing of the sentence. Everybody wants to be part of the miracle and witnessing improvements on a daily basis they seize their opportunity to make a difference. What a wonderful human characteristic.

I feel I have run my miles in a muddy marathon and regrettably must 'Pass on the Baton', but I can pass with love and advice to help him tackle his tricky miles to come.

PJ Care has enabled me to be at his side during this early stage and although the challenges may differ, the grit and determination he will need are the same.

He has stacks!

I watched him eating an Easter egg

"What are we celebrating Curtis?"

From behind chocolate covered lips

He replies

"LIFE!"

-Thank god for the gift of laughter-

(Lost Blueprints – Memories)

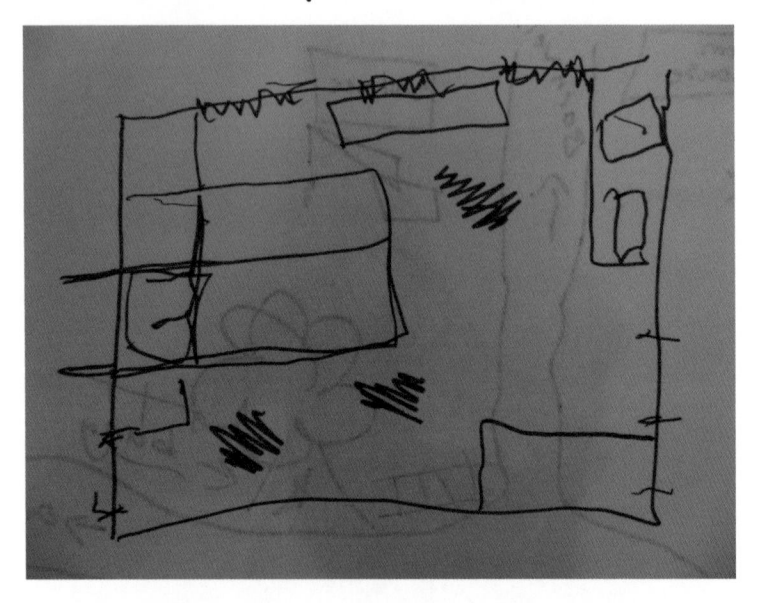

Mine Top – Families bottom

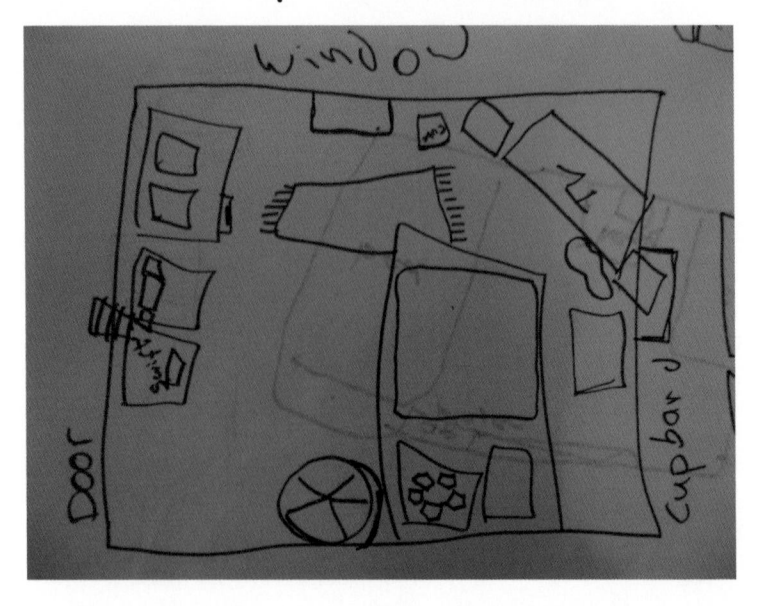

My Conclusion

Working with different abilities, studying mannerisms, behaviour and body language over the years has lead me to a few conclusions about my own phsycological and physical movements.

We are all creatures of our experiences that make up our actions, memories and therefore our knowledge. You know what you can remember.

Through talking with close family about my ABI, I have found myself unsettled with their view that I misread signs and situations of daily occurrence, somehow miss the obvious which leads me to respond inappropriately via comment or joke.

We all have a perception of how our actions affect other people and adjust our behaviour accordingly. A proportion of this is missing in me and has been pointed out as being a crack in my character. The most unnerving thing is, I can't see it and feel no need for change.

I know of two people who have been Sectioned due to brain damage and have met hundreds of people whose brains have not fully developed and I find them both familiar and easy company.

I have worked with some wonderful people with Autism and Asperger's Syndrome, the connection comes when you start to relate with the many similarities between the habits of your damaged brain and their needs.

Cognitive Behaviour Therapy (CBT) is a psychotherapeutic approach that addresses dysfunctional emotions and behaviours. Our cognitive processes are our thoughts, which include our ideas, mental images, beliefs and attitudes.

In my Preface I stated that I was convinced my family had been approached by phycotherapists, to help tackle any problems I may be left with.

CBT can help you make sense of problems by breaking them down into smaller parts. Your thoughts, feelings, physical sensations and actions are interconnected, each one can affect the others. For example, your thoughts about a problem can often affect how you feel both physically and emotionally, as well as how you act on the problem. Negative thought cycles lead to many unwanted cognitive patterns within your brain.

CBT was directly inspired by ancient Greek philosophy. Socrates, Plato and Aristotle. This proves to me that what Tom was feeling and seeing was right after Jerry's actions. Brain damage feels very personal and individual but people have experienced it since the dawn of time.

I do not hold on to clutter in my brain, being weighed down by any negative thoughts for a day and they are forgotten by the following morning. This has its benefits but makes lessons harder to learn.

"Who can discover without a Lesson Learnt?"

It is a human characteristic to climb the tree of life only striving to reach the ripest of fruit that are better than the rest. Meaning of course there is always better to be found no matter what your circumstances are. Your mind is always stretched reaching for the better 'scrump'. This characteristic has been suppressed in me like my immune system due to drugs, to control my autoimmune condition.

I am very happy with the bruised fruit at the bottom that others would not even consider. My mind is wandering around a 99p store picking up thoughts, feelings and fruit that seem to be a bargain at the time.

I am a lot more susceptible to thought however unreasonable or irrelevant, becoming lost in it for minutes lasting days.

I have a lack of self-consciousness or as I prefer to call it, confidence and am socially hot and cold in random patterns completely out of my hands.

When explaining things or expressing myself, often it will take me a good few goes at getting to the point, if ever!

Once more I find myself ducking and diving over and under all descriptive words trying to hit the bulls eye, (make my point). This process is called circumlocution, the use of too many words.

Expressive aphasia in cognitive neurophysiology happens when you damage specific parts of the brain and may hamper your ability to produce language, spoken or written.

Now we have just tapped into another set of lasting problems I was left with. I struggle with the detailed task of writing, processing my thoughts into the letter shapes then the words, takes time.

I have written a few helpful lists for people suffering the lasting effects of an ABI. My approach to writing, reading and speaking is as follows:

Writing

1. Pause and breath before starting, concentration is the key - focus!
2. Think of a letter shape, picture it BIG!
3. Press pen firmly on paper, by pushing down you will have more control over direction, it will also help stop you jumping two steps forward and scribbling.
4. Copy your simple letter shape keeping to a larger scale.

DO NOT start small and fail.

5. Pull the pen away after each letter.
6. Re-focus and picture the next.

One letter at – a - time.

Perhaps try leaving b i g   g a p s, as a way of helping you breath. I find lower case easier!

Reading

1. Pause, focus eyes, maybe blink a couple of times. You may suffer with double vision.

2. Read the first word slowly and out loud. This will not only enable you to keep pronunciation and clarity, but give your mind time to process/understand.

3. Move through one word at a time, at a slow pace.

4. Do not move on till the word you are reading is fully understood and its relation to words preceding it in the sentence.

4. If ever in doubt, go back and read it again, it will take time to process. I often read a whole sentence and have not understood a word in it.

5. I use a blank sheet of paper for a bookmark, writing down page numbers, as I never trust where I finished. Also this is handy for writing notes, which are essential to my understanding of the book.

Speaking

1. Think about what you want to say.

2. Say it through in your head, maybe highlighting possible hurdles.

3. Pause, breath, start to speak loudly and clearly. One word at – a – time.

4. Break up your sentence as much as you can. Your mind may focus on the end of the sentence, this will only make you speed up.

5. After every word, stop, and think where your sentence is going, so not to get lost in words.

6. And finally your voice may be fairly flat, so try focusing on the punctuation of your sentence. Practice makes perfect, try reading in your room without the pressure of expectation, putting into practice methods that work for you. Some days will be better then others, noise levels are key to my ability.

Knowing all this (as if possessed by 'Road Runner'), I still scribble the last word of a sentence in an obscene hurry. Distraction in as little as a thought ruins all the concentration I can muster.

My speech slurs and I process information slowly. When I am tired or the effort is not there for one reason or another you will be lucky to understand a single word I say, as if I loose control of my own mind for a second. It sends me shooting off in the wrong direction at the wrong pace.

Headway have helped me talk to other people who's brains are still re-booting, finishing each others sentences as if in a club, a kind of members only way.

This does not feel right?

I should have landed somewhere else!

With ideas flowing and similarities a plenty, I find myself in a world I was not born into and it scares me. Not the concept, just that I am a new person with a new heading.

Although my damaged brain is lacking activity in some areas, energy has been re-directed to a previously unused part of brain and awoken somebody who never should have existed.

This somebody is easy company, he takes things at his own selfish pace and will not slow down on request. He will make time for people on his own terms.

His most redeeming features are his ability to emotionally connect with others and their situations.

I am here and can only live life to the best of my own knowledge. I do not have any particular drive or goals, however I do remember saying.

"It was much easier to let each day drift by"

A part of my mind is still lost in empty space. I do try to drift in the right direction, an estimated guess of where I want to be while my brain continues to re-program.

My ever so excited friend
Text: "Luckily your recovery precipitated new discoveries"

"Life is all about how you feel inside"
"It is wonderful to be alive!"

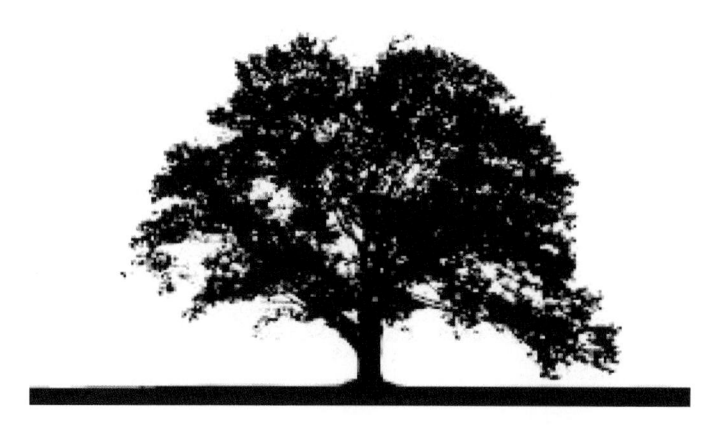

Rehab to Rehab
Working with PJ Care and looking from the inside out

POSTSCRIPT:

I recently hit the proverbial 'nail on the head' when speaking to a nurse at PJ Care. I told her the reason for my success with understanding the patients at work is due to looking from the inside-out having been in their situation, as opposed to a qualified professional looking from the outside in.

Seeing things through a neurological patients eye's is especially important. Understanding their journey is crucial to understanding the path that lies before them.

They will range in mental capacity so being able to understand feelings and emotions that they may have, along with years of experience working with mentally handicapped people, has helped me offer the best of me.

Lets re-cap the lasting effects of an ABI and the challenges it leaves in its wake. Most people overlook how complex a life becomes when the psychological setbacks for an acquired brain injury victim become a day to day struggle, completing the mundane tasks that are essential to living in a hectic modern world in a rush or a hurry.

From personal care, eating your breakfast, to work with lunch breaks, meetings, conducting yourself, speaking, writing, endlessly giving silent signals though body language and returning home to a social life, eating a meal while socializing with loved ones in some capacity.

Think of all the movements, physical and phsycological that go un-witnessed by the human eye. Every millisecond of every day a remarkable string of events occurs in the human brain! Billions of brain cells called neurons transmit signals to each other and they do it at trillions of junctions called synapses. Many acted without your knowing or say so.

So subtle like an ant working his way through the most complex of alarm systems, light sensors and touch sensitive bells on his way home.

No trouble at all, with the ant being next to weightless and smaller than a thimble!

Socializing covers everything from a glance in the street to making love, communicating through body language to the word, written or spoken. When taken away or changed though it can alter your friend-making skills or finding a partner. These are surely our given rights, a signed document written and stamped at each and every birth guaranteeing some sort of life to be lived?

Life teaches us one by one in many different ways respect and not to expect anything.

Writing, reading and walking are basic life skills of which you only fully understand as being necessary when they have been lost for minutes or days.

Months or years, the effects of brain damage can be for life. Forever stuck with them until you pass on. So the sooner you can adapt, adjust and accept them, your quality of life will be better.

Here again are the possible effects of brain damage;

- Cognitive effects
- Coma and reduced awareness states
- Communication problems
- Emotional and behavioral effects
- Executive dysfunction
- Hormonal imbalances and pituitary dysfunction
- Post traumatic amnesia (PTA)
- Vegetative states

I am with my fourth Renault Clio. The point is that ever since my crash in 2003, the one that left many phsycological and physical impairments left me striving to find my previous normal self, even though it was never going to be the normal I had been accustomed to. The quality of life that had been taken for granted was now a dream that belonged in the clouds.

Ever striving to reach my optimal potential was mainly done on my own, physiotherapists can only help you reach a stage, after that it relies on your hard work and persistence to gain a recovery that enables you to carry on.

Everything back in its place like playing a game of dominos, lining up a complex course winding and carving for nineteen years. Then starting the game with a wrong push! Recovery being when you're slowly rebuilding the course one by one, the painstaking task of lifting them all back up onto their feet. The last nineteen years, even one a day would mean 6930 dominos, some more out of place then others, but all needing adjustment to be anywhere near their last position.

Somewhere between the playful act of letting your mind wander and drifting off to a pleasant state of thought, suddenly the game becomes a fight for life that would last a lifetime at some level.

My second Renault Clio – As soon as I was able I was signed into a contract by Renault, who would take near on two hundred pounds from my bank account in return for a brand new Clio, in black of course! I needed it to be as close to the last as possible, the latest, shiny, new, glossy, air-conditionined, electric windows etc. Not quite enough room to swing a cat, but spacious and unlike my first, clean! I was back on the road, continuing my journey from Polebrook to Thrapston from Oundle.

Listen, you don't for one minute think they would let somebody back on the road after brain damage without taking an eye test do you? Oh no, I had to read a number plate from a good few yards of which I pulled out of the bag on my third and final attempt, YES!

It was just another evening, being winter there was a low and blinding sun. It was a Friday after a hot, sweaty, sticky day in the sweet factory and the time was 5.30 approx. I am ashamed to say I had a 4 minutes drive home from work but after a minute, as I pulled away from the sweet factory I drove for two seconds unable to see due to the sun.

In or on the 'second' second I ploughed into Paddy's wife's parked car on the road outside the factory. Luckily my speed did not exceed 5 miles per hour or this would be a different story.

An apology, shake of hands with the exchange of a few documents and my shameful four-minute drive home looking out of my window, over the smashed bonnet was my punishment. I got off lightly with Paddy's wife being sat in the parked car!

I cannot even begin to say how bad I felt. Concentration was there but sometimes, as this story demonstrates, it is not enough to stop an accident.

The rush of modern life often leads to a lack of caution, in no way is it an excuse, but it is a reality.

I drove to GERMANY a few years back, something I'm very proud to have done, what with them on the wrong side and all, once again a whole new mindset to the perception of the road system.

Anybody who has driven in Europe and other such places with this back to front approach, will possible have adapted almost instantly, however I had it in only a little outside of this time frame, but boy was it worth it. I found myself looking at sights concerning a more tragic subject - The Great War!

Gazing over the many thousands of head stones wondering how many were due to head injures that were unable to be treated and again considering how they would have been tackled with the historic medical knowledge they had between 1914 - 1918

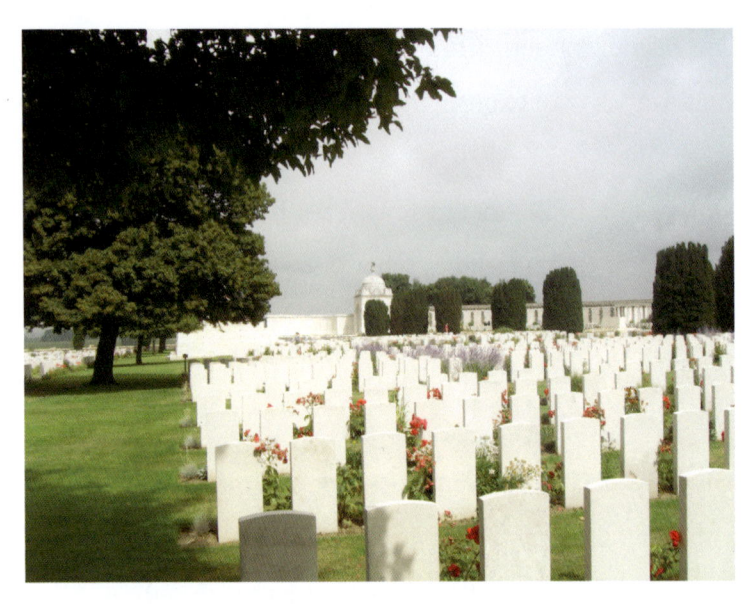

An iconic view from Tyne Cott cemetery

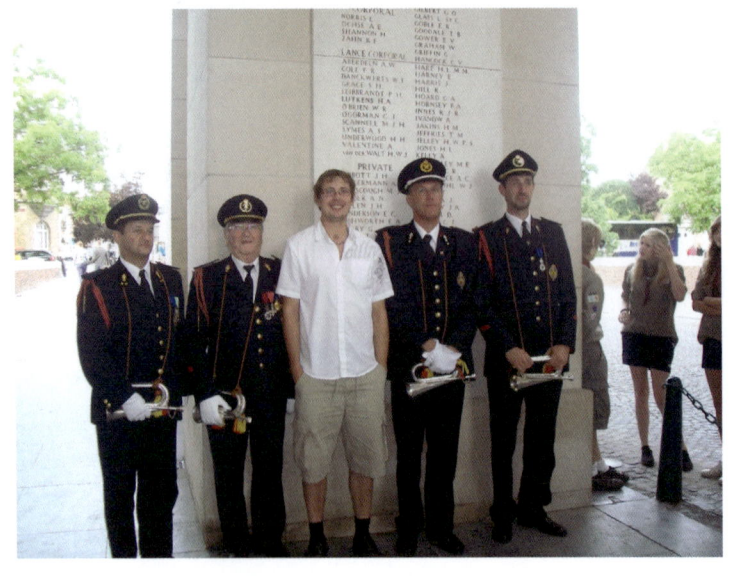

Ypres: last post at the Menin Gate

Like many others I am lucky to live in an age of rapid medical advances. Because of the efforts of thousands of medical scientists around the world who are indirectly making life safer to live unlike the soldiers then going over the top to almost certain death.

Lets go back to playing dominos of pre-existence, all 6930 of them counting for every day I was on the original route I was born into. Each one represents a characteristic, mannerism, mood, expression or path of thought.

We know the brain is plastic and malleable and we know that it can strengthen and improve with experience, practice and determination. So re-carving my neurological pathways was inevitable.

This means the normal I have found differs from the previous normal that had felt so comfy with where I would be able to drift in and out of concentration and re-focusing would take seconds.

Unfortunately concentration as far as I am aware has been the key to its demise. I am unable to pull in and out of concentration with as little as a thought any more. It takes the right environment; sounds are key to my ability. Distraction is an evil killer when in the wrong hands.

My third Renault Clio – Ok, so I've had some painful memories in Clio's, not always being held on to like a space man in a suit or a boy freewheeling on his bike, but they do seem to be my - I hate to use the word again – Destiny? Shiny, air-conditioning, electric windows and enough room to swing a cat, in a nice bright sporty metallic blue!

Now if this is not a fresh start I don't know what is. I had an extra beam of light that would turn on, as if sent from - God - as I turned particularly challenging corners.

The conditions I knew were wet. I was pressed for time, got it. I had in the last week replaced my tyres, fully aware. I had not, for one reason or another focussed. The A14 roundabout would remind me of all these things as if I had set my alarm clock to shock!

The new tyres inevitably slid and being a roundabout of course gravity thought it would have a dig too. The car rolled, like there were no other influences, and we landed safely but shook up 360 degrees later.

I forgot to tell you about the impressive six air bag capacity which all blew up like party balloons, in seconds. None of the air bags got their chance to be the hero as thankfully they were not needed, like the footballer sat in shirt number 12 on the bench all alone secretly wishing a team mate would have 'the cramp', so that he would be able to shine, play his game with prospects of being chosen for his first cap for England.

I opened the door, with a push mind you, to stumble out and stagger a few paces in case the director called for an explosion throwing me up into the air, the car blowing up pushing me a further 10 yards into a bush.

The immediate reaction was to call my brother. He lives nearby and in hearing my crashed car statement, he replied, knowing of previous incidents, you're joking aren't you?

He turned up along with the police and an ambulance to a queue of traffic tragically long, if you were involved I can only apologise. The incident shows you how thin the paper is between an accident and tragedy.

I believe it was after this particular event that I was reminded of a little talk between Richard my barber and myself. He told me, boys especially won't learn after one mistake but that it would take several knocks, like trying to attach a fridge magnet to a wooden fridge.

The human brain has varying strengths of magnetism, some hold their sign up like at a college rally, others did not even turn up.

My fourth Renault Clio – I have been with the same black, 08 plate Renault Clio since 2008. Many people have complimented me on my driving being safe and feeling comfortable. Possibly because of my anticipation of an accident round every corner as there has been in the past.

When learning to drive you become obsessed with the A to B, focusing on the B and almost picturing yourself sitting in B. This will speed you up and becomes a distraction from the hundreds of hurdles you need to jump in order to reach B, never mind sitting. This is something I have little choice over now and have re-learnt to – BREATHE.

Of course it gets forgotten occasionally otherwise I would be perfect. We all know the only thing perfect in the world is the colonel's recipe for chicken.

Near on every year I have been able to drive to Wales, it's worth being alive for I promise you. You can be in the clouds and an hour later you can be wearing a crash helmet with a torch down, The Big Pit.

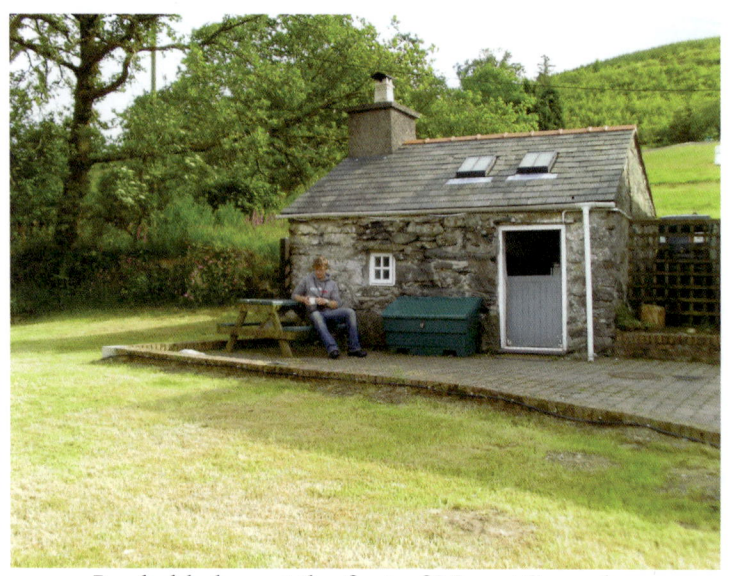

Lockable box at the foot of Mount Snowdon

I think my post (statement), on the internet struck a cord with people, thank you again for such wonderful encouragement to try something new, explore my life in a way that makes you think about every word, one word at – a - time if your typing is anything like mine.

PJ Care
specialised neurological care

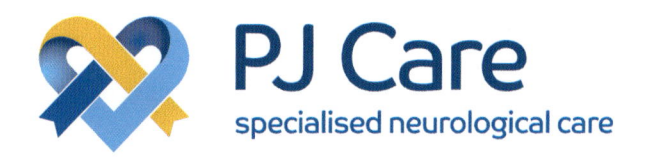

Since starting at PJ Care in November 2013, ten years after my crash, I have seen some amazing improvements, people jumping so many hurdles like Aries Merritt (USA) London 2012. However you will need patience as any improvement from a Neurological condition can take a lifetime.

On employment you will be enriched with these responsibilities to guide you though this journey of discovery and help you to lead your mind though the tricky neurological challenges you will face.

Summary of responsibilities.

Participating as a full member of the nursing team in the assessing, planning, implementation, and evaluation of individual care plans.

To assist senior care staff working with other agencies and professionals ensuring full provision of individual residents care.

Provide ongoing monitoring, support and assessment of residents physical and phsycological and social needs.

Assist in the induction of new care staff
Provide support and supervision of care staff as delegated by the registered nurse on duty.

To follow company policies and procedures at all times and to relate to relatives and carers with empathy.

To attend mandatory training courses relevant to the position at the direction of your manager.

All of this has helped stretch my mind to reconnect like a recoiling strap, so frustrating to attach, but essential to holding things in place.

Let us think about giving neurologically challenged people a boost to a level of recovery.

Training, education and more importantly recovery is found everywhere, goal orientated objectives to complete with a deadline for motivation. College courses, home courses to playtime and building colour coordinated blocks. Going over the many topics more than once is essential. This may need to be done regularly as memory strength may vary.

Working with PJ Care has reminded me of these things time and time again as other target based tasks in social skills, camaraderie, and more practical duties like moving and handling at a steady pace. Just think of 'Pacman', slowly carving out new Nero-pathways.

Following the sometimes patronising training taking you back to the start has helped me back up onto my feet. Bending at the knees and keeping good posture are the details I know we all partly forget over time, unless reminded. Handicapped people are reminded every day!

Handicapped is such a derogatory term but describes more people than the first thought suggests.

A closed head injury leaves you mentally handicapped on some level like the man wearing a number 12 shirt who is on as substitute wearing two left boots, at first glimpse he appears absolutely fine and healthy but when he tries to run on the disability becomes apparent.

On recruitment with PJ Care you will undertake a series of essential courses to remind you of the basics, good practise and some vital new information to help you administer the best possible care, but you are the main piece of therapy equipment these people have.

Interaction is very important; you can try playing any kind of game or just chatting to them, both equally beneficial and both equally rewarding. Family is important but not essential. The benefits of family can be familiarity and memories, long and short term.

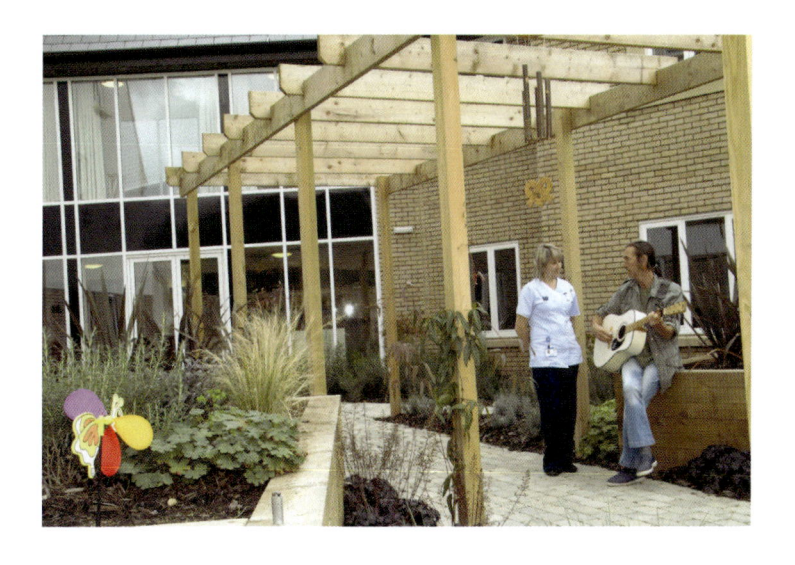

Memory triggers can be directly posed questions or more subtle talk to establish where their memory lies. Familiar places, people and activities may send off a firework in their mind.

Remember it may take time to look for that tiny book/memory in the world's largest library, your mind!

Since being driven to the best recovery since Spurs came from 4-0 down to a 4-4 victory, I have had the freedom to fly like a bird to Devon, Ireland, Brecon Beacons and Germany etc.

PJ Neurological Care is my best placement to date. I am making the most of my freedom with sights I am so glad to be alive to see, Giant's Causeway in Ireland, Temple Mount in Jerusalem and other amazing places.

My change in career has lead me to be part of amazing social events that without my determination to beat the stubborn other team would have been impossible.

Without this found again freedom I would have had to find magic and all of my life's joy in the light at the end of the tunnel I would have been living in, a very secluded affair.

This type of life is not the end by any means, it may be a steeper hill with more rocks but the human mind I am sure can overcome, jump any hurdle, if the conditions are favourable.

If the capacity is not there, the victory may take a combined effort of family and friends to keep their fire alight. All concerned will need a positive outlook.

I appreciate keeping your own log pile stocked can be hard at times. You will need to wander deep into a possibly dark, cold and scary forest in order to gather enough wood to drive you both through the early days and beyond. It will not be a brisk walk after an ABI and will test and drive the patience of everybody concerned.

PJ Care prints a monthly magazine, 'The Script', full of exciting new progress made by the professionals and importantly the HCA's who are fundamental to the overall progress on any of the units at Eglewood in Peterborough.

Humanism is a system of values and beliefs that is based on the idea that people are basically good and that problems can be solved using reason instead of religion, i.e, Living your life in other peoples shoes.

Seeing things through eyes of which may be alien to you and not just seeing but understanding their ideas, beliefs and their likes and dislikes.

All of which is crucial to making up their actions, not forgetting their history which also must be understood as it animates and defines who they were and who they will be as long as they are here and living the present.

I fully understand everybody has different sized feet and choice of shoe is also to be considered. Like your personality some have a big, bold, brightly coloured shoe while others will favour a pastel coloured shoe with a subtle design. People's thoughts work in very much the same way. People may be quiet but they have big plans, ideas to change the world or their footwear if they're wearing thin!

Example:

A patient who had travelled the world, owned a business, had worked hard throughout their life and had children, now grown up.

They have a stroke that leaves spasticity and contracture down one side of their body, continually experiencing pain and anxiety.

Entering their room you would be mindful of their night's sleep of which will determine the mood and path of conversation. Waiting for the patient's reactions to determine how much pain he or she may or may not be in.

A comfortable and a spacious look should be left in a room of rest for individuality to be stamped to suit the phsycological needs of any patient who rests there for a period of time.

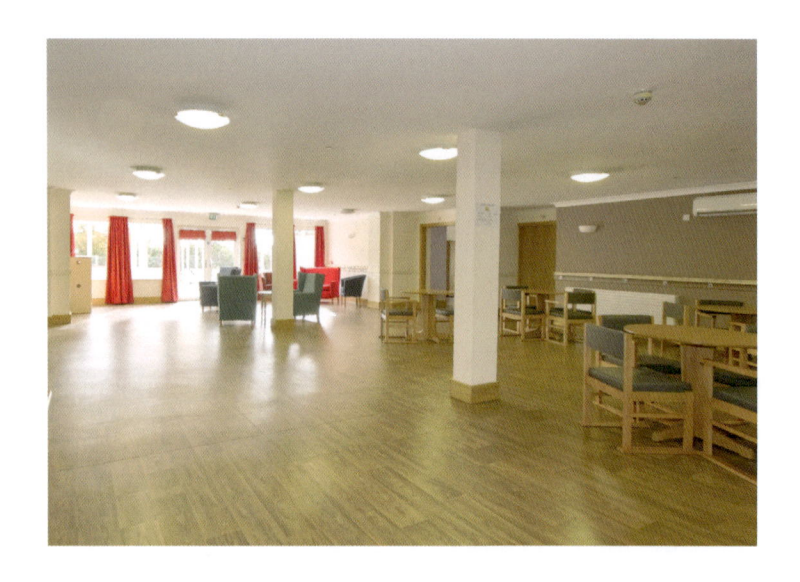

Respite, winter bed or a stay for which most definitely needs a feeling of home, an ideal setting for an open mind to start to fill with positive memories and information.

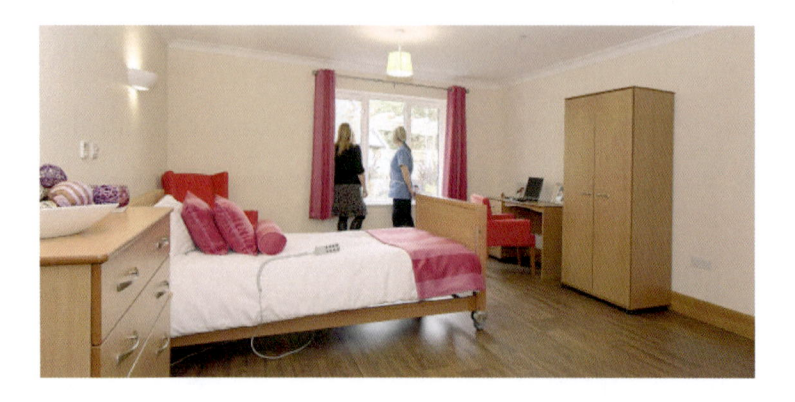

I am now wearing the patient's shoes, being sympathetic to their every concern. Imagining a hampered lifestyle while considering how they, not I, would like to be spoken to and treated on this one of many different mornings.

You should positively stimulate minds with old memories they possess of their past or brand new positive topics about the days to come, not drifting into dreams or guessing the future.

If possible do not quiz them in the morning but at a settled time in the afternoon. I would pose questions about any travelling, avoiding possible negative memories.

We know positivity is a healer you cannot have too much, but be selective of when and where you apply it by judging the mood of the room. By increasing activity in the brain you are training and giving it plenty of experience. This is the main way to increase chances of a draw in the football match. It may strengthen and improve that which already exists.

Engage them in lots of social activity even if this means going to your local coffee shop and people watching, this is not only a step back to normality but it helps them become aware once more of peoples natural actions and reactions.

Perhaps copy and paste them in their own story like a newborn, taken on board like a mass of holidaymakers setting off on a cruise of life.

A goal that any acquired brain damage or Stroke victim wishes to score is the equalizer that puts them on level terms. Places them back in the game where anything is possible. At least giving them a fighting chance of a win.

Set backs are hard to swallow a whole new mindset is required.

Many patients I work with spend a lot of time in a state of frustration with their new capabilities being different to the previous that had felt so comfy.

Making a cup of tea or brushing your teeth are intolerable tasks when unable to process the movement (Dyspraxia) let alone the task.

The people you will encounter may be new to disability so be patient, they also, in many cases expect a full recovery.

A mistake on neurological wards would be doing things to the patient the way you would like it to be done to you. The patient has different capacity than you and may or may not be struggling with their own thoughts. At times you must wear those hard to fit shoes!

Their history can be learnt though reading care plans as well as hearing stories of their pre-incident life in their own words to understand where they are neurologically.

This is the best way to meet their needs, not using your self as the model, but wearing the models shoes.

Hypochondriacs can be bed ridden for weeks with nothing more then a mild pain which chips away at the bone in their mind, slowly carving its way through neurological pathways finding more pain which may or may not be there. Stumbling across other problems which may disturb your previously stable mind-set, magnifying any stress or anxiety to massive levels that stops the body receiving positive information from the brain.

Chemical imbalances and traumatic life experiences such as a head injury may contribute to the development of hypochondria.

The only reason I mention it is because of a neuron carrying the wrong negative message can detrimentally affect the body and mind. This leads to an unhealthy outlook.

Psychotherapy such as cognitive behavior therapy (CBT) and behavioural stress management can be effective in treating hypochondria as well as other conditions, which may arise.

This involves regular counseling with a psychotherapist to recognize false beliefs, understand anxiety, and stop anxious behaviours. Lowering negative thought cycles and positivity are essential to their lives, to keep the score 0-0.

PJ sponsors a local rugby team and took part in a corporate rugby match with teams such as Jaguar, Landrover. We went along with patients of neurology.

This is an activity that thousands of patients would benefit from all over the UK, a social, visually driven, outdoor activity.

PJ won and the patients came onto the pitch, had photos taken and were very much part of the day, involved! Each was given a PJ rugby top and enjoyed the ride home with smiles to show off back in Peterborough.

A racehorse at the Grand National with its shiny coat, muscles to achieve its habits and needs to fulfil its every potential, has been groomed and fed energy and exercised for years to accomplish a win.

We hamper the senses by making the horse wear blinkers giving it tunnel vision, thereby focussing its eyesight on the B or finish line. This speeds him up as we discussed earlier. Cancelling any distraction from the task in hand whether it be reading, writing, speaking, driving over a roundabout or winning the race.

If we think about the hurdles as being social interactions, Christmases, wedding anniversaries, baptisms, football matches, passing your driving test, or buying a new home and breaking them all down to the movements involved along with associated feelings - you will see life.

After an ABI or stroke you can live your life with a very intense view of the world focussing on the one subject endlessly, tunnel vision or, what I like to call, tunnel thought for hours.

When out of the dark woods where you had been gathering love, sensation, taste, acceptance and emotion, with training and experience hopefully you can return to a more spacious, enlightened view of the world, your course of dominos will almost be reset.

I wish everybody peace and happiness.

    Life is about the journey, not the destination….

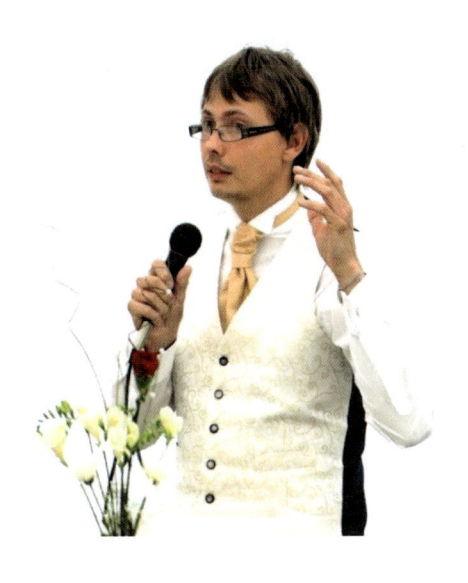

"I must thank Stephen for allowing us to accompany him on his journey. This is a wonderful read that really highlights brain injury from the patient's perspective.

The journey is a helter skelter ride through Stephen's thought processes and absolutely riveting at every point. I was unable to put it down, reading from cover to cover twice.

Stephen tells a great tale and a really heart warming one. I am proud that we have been a part of his journey, Stephen has brought a fresh perspective to me and to his colleagues and I hope that everyone who has any kind of involvement with brain injury reads this and takes his message to heart."

Neil Russell
Chief Operating Officer - PJ Care Ltd.

"Rehab to Rehab is a wonderful read if you want to understand what life is like with a brain injury. Stephen's writing is truly poetic and quirky. More to the point, it is a very real insight for anyone who knows someone with a brain injury, or if they work in neurological rehabilitation. Thank you Stephen for bringing a fresh perspective to acquired brain injury"

Mary Goode
Chief Executive, Headway Cambridgeshire

This is the ongoing story of one individual. There are thousands of journeys starting every year with such varied challenges. Never judge people on behaviour or mentality alone, take time to understand their journey, overlooked by many including me, but please keep trying.

ACKNOWLADGEMENT

The Author greatly appreciates the efforts of all the dedicated trained staff, family, friends, Headway and PJ Specialist neurological care

Dedicated to families suffering for a *loved* one.

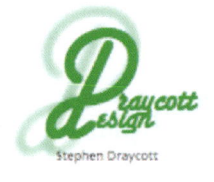

Draycott Design
Stephen Draycott

draycottdesign@gmail.com

DO YOU HAVE A BRAIN INJURY OR KNOW SOMEONE WHO HAS?

Headway Cambridgeshire can help. We provide a range of activities, some free, some for a small fee and some using your personal budget.

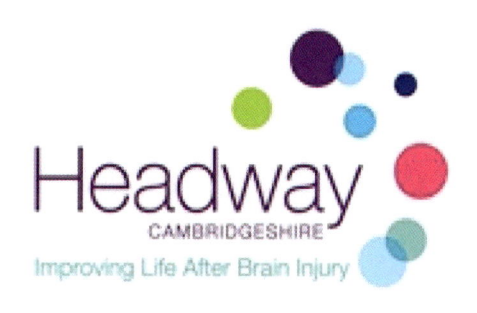

STRUCTURED SOCIAL REHABILITATION

Hub Programmes

Our Hubs in and Peterborough offer a programme of activities aimed at recovery and social rehabilitation following brain injury. We provide a supportive and therapeutic environment where individual needs, skills and contributions are valued. Individuals can choose from a range of sessions which will support their individual goals. This could be building physical fitness and stamina, improving daily living skills, increasing your social network, understanding and managing the effects of your injury or improving your wellbeing

To find out what we can offer, or for an assessment, contact Kathy Bullock on 01223 576550 or email kathyb@headway-cambs.org.uk

MOTIVATIONAL/GOAL SETTING COURSES

We run motivational courses tailored to meet the specific learning needs of people living with a brain injury (ie memory, concentration, processing and fatigue). Courses promote goal setting, skills development and health improvement.

Wisbech/Peterborough Contact Carole McNeill on 01733 616070 or email carolem@headway-cambs.org.uk

Cambridge/Papworth Contact Clare Hobbs on 01223 576550 or clareh@headway-cambs.org.uk

INFORMATION, ADVICE & SUPPORT

Our Brain Injury Co-ordinators are here to offer information, advice and support to anyone affected by brain injury at any point.

Examples of support we can give include:

* Information on brain injury

* Information on Headway Services

* Information on other services across Cambridgeshire

* Benefits support

* Signposting to relevant agencies

* Emotional support

We are happy to talk through a range of issues via telephone or in person at one of our hubs, at your home or at Addenbrooke's hospital. Contact Jo on 01223 576550 (Cambridgeshire), Sharon on 01733 516070 (Peterborough), Catherine 01223 256018

COMMUNITY ENABLEMENT/REHABILITATION

Our Independence service provides specialist rehabilitation workers to help you to achieve your goals at home or in the community. The types of support we could provide include:

* Re-ablement following discharge from hospital or residential services

* Support with daily living

* Support to build confidence in community facilities

* Support to engage in social, learning or volunteer opportunities

* Support to manage effects of brain injury

Contact Nicola on 01223 576550 or email nicolah@headway-cambs.org.uk

ART THERAPY

Following a brain injury you may have experienced many changes to your life. Art Therapy gives you the chance to use art materials to express thoughts and feelings that are difficult to talk about. You do not need to be good at art to come; all ages and abilities are welcome.

Contact Clare on 01223 576550 or email clareh@headway-cambs.org.uk to learn more about art therapy or book your session.

HORTICULTURAL THERAPY

Plants, wildlife and green space have always played an important role in helping people to recover from physical and psychological ailments. At Headway, we have created a great new, accessible therapy garden where you can join our gardening group to grow fruit and veg in our poly tunnel and raised beds, enjoy the beautiful wildlife, flowers and trees, and help take care of our friendly chickens. Sessions are run on Tuesdays and Fridays with our trained horticultural therapist and cover a range of activities throughout the year.

Contact Simon on 01223 576550 or email simonl@headway-cambs.org.uk to find out more.

OCCUPATIONAL THERAPY

We provide specialist assessment and input to support your goals with the aim of improving or maintaining function and independence. Areas where our Occupational Therapist might be able to help you include:

* Support for learning, training or work

* Approaches and strategies to help with daily living

* Effective techniques and practical advice for managing cognitive or emotional difficulties

* Support and advice in relation to adaptive equipment

Contact Nicola on 01223 576550 or email nicolah@headway-cambs.org.uk to find out more

LEISURE

Open Gym on Mondays

We have a great gym at our hub in Fulbourn which we are opening up so anyone can use it from 10am – 2.30pm on Mondays, so if you would like to get fitter in a safe and gentle environment come along. Whatever age you are, whether or not you have a disability, you will have great support from our gym instructor, Veer.

Contact Veer on 01223 576550 or email veerd@headway-cambs.org.uk to learn more about our gym or book your session

ALLOTMENT - CAMBRIDGE

Our thriving community allotment, just off Coldham's Lane in Cambridge, provides a great opportunity to socialise in the fresh air, get fit, grow your own fruit and veg and enjoy a well-earned cuppa and a chat in the potting shed at the end of the day. It doesn't matter whether you are a seasoned gardener who knows their onions, or whether you are a total novice who doesn't don't know an aubergine from a carrot - you are always welcome at the Headway allotment. Sessions run on Tuesdays and Fridays all year round.

Contact Simon on 01223 576550 or email simonl@headway-cambs.org.uk to find out more.

YOUTH

Headway Youth is a vibrant, fun, supportive group for young people aged 16-25 (ish). We are a friendly, welcoming bunch who do all sorts of social activities from tenpin bowling to graffiti, socials to activity days. In Cambridge we meet fortnightly on Wednesday evenings, 7-9pm, the venue changes depending on what we are doing. Come along to get some peer support, amake some new friends and try out some fun activities.

Contact John on 01223 576550 or email johnp@headway-cambs.org.uk

ABOUT US

Headway Cambridgeshire is a registered charity that provides a range of services designed to meet the needs of clients, families and anybody supporting people with a brain injury or neurological condition.

We recognise that clients and family members need appropriate support and services to enable them to make positive changes in their lives. We have a strong ethos of promoting independence and a 'can do' approach that provides flexible, client focused solutions that leave people feeling supported and able to move on.

If you have any questions at all, ring us on 01223 576550 or email info@headway-cambs.org.uk

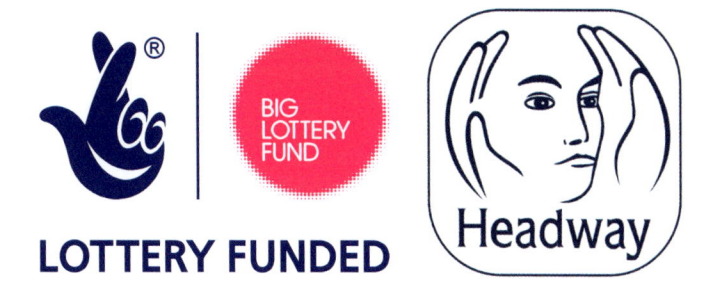